AFTER CANCER
Now What?

A *Biblical Guide* to Navigating Life After Cancer

THERESIA WHITFIELD

LUCIDBOOKS

After Cancer: Now What?
A Biblical Guide to Navigating Life After Cancer
Copyright © 2025 by Theresia Whitfield

Published by Lucid Books in Houston, TX
www.LucidBooks.com

ISBN: 978-1-63296-903-3
eISBN: 978-1-63296-848-7

Special Sales: Most Lucid Books titles are available in special quantity discounts. Custom imprinting or excerpting can also be done to fit special needs. Contact Lucid Books at Info@LucidBooks.com

For my husband, Kurt, whose love and support in seeing my dreams come true have never wavered.

TABLE OF CONTENTS

INTRODUCTION

One person's cancer journey is not the same as someone else's. If that's true, why am I bothering to tell you about my journey? It's because I want to give you, the reader, a glimpse into the life of someone who has traversed this difficult road. This book takes a real, hard, raw look into what I went through. It isn't to toot my own horn or show how wonderful I am because I did this. I take heart with this scripture:

> *I know how to be brought low, and I know how to abound. In any and every circumstance, I have learned the secret of facing plenty and hunger, abundance and need. I can do all things through him who strengthens me.*
>
> —Phil. 4:12–13

Cancer is not an easy battle. If you're in the middle of it, you already know this. But for those reading this book who might have a loved one facing this battle, I want you to see how difficult it can be—not to frighten you but rather to encourage you. I believe it's important to have a concept of what someone with cancer goes through on their journey.

If a loved one is going through a cancer journey, know that they need you. They may not admit it at first, if ever, but they need you to be there for them. They need someone stable in their world of chaos—and yes, it will be full of chaos at times. They need someone to encourage them. They need you to pray for them and with them without ceasing. In Chapter 8, I talk about faith and community—how they are necessary for victory in the battle against cancer. You are part of that circle. Stay there no matter how ugly it gets. And it *will* get ugly. Simply stay there.

If you've already been through this journey, I want you to see that you have not struggled alone or struggled in vain. I tell my story to encourage you. You and I both made it by the grace of God. And I want you to know you are not alone in what you are experiencing in the aftermath of your cancer journey.

If you're new to this journey, I want you to know that I am here for you. This is one person's story—my story—and it likely won't be exactly what you experience, even if you have the same type of cancer I had. People respond differently to chemotherapy, radiation, and surgery. Some people fly right through the journey with little more than an external scar. Praise God! Some struggle mightily. I did. And I want you to see it for its realness and rawness, to remind you that if I can do it, so can you. I want to remind you that God is faithful. Even when we can't trace His hand, we can always trust His heart.

A couple of months after my mastectomy, I began to struggle with the psychological trauma of having survived cancer. I realized that I had looked death in the face. I could have died. God chose to save me and heal me, and I'm grateful. But it shook me to the core. I wasn't sure how to deal with it.

Not long after that, I started wondering how to navigate life after cancer. I had free time now. No longer were my days filled with appointments, labs, scans, chemotherapy, physical therapy, and other cancer-related things. What would I do with all this free time? Yes, I was back to co-leading a small group with my husband, Kurt, and our friends. And yes, I was back facilitating our women's Bible study at church. But it was so rote. I was simply going through the motions. I was starting to feel better physically, so no one was visiting me anymore. Everyone had moved on with their lives. I was growing hair, dealing with three-month checkups with my oncologist, and sometimes having scans, which always frightened me. And I didn't know what to do with my extra time.

During my cancer journey—all the chemo and surgeries—every second of every single day had been dictated by infusions, labs, follow-up shots, sleep, nausea, doctors' appointments, and scans. There wasn't time for me to live my own life or process the emotions I was having. That was my life. Then the treatments were over, and the cancer was gone. Suddenly, I was free. Now what?

I started searching for books on the subject of navigating life after cancer, wondering how to get back some semblance of normalcy. I found a few books, but they were very secular and insisted on taking the bull by the horns and empowering yourself.

I knew those ideals were at odds with my Christian faith that teaches me that my strength comes from the Lord, not within me alone. God alone is my strength and my song. As the scripture says, "I can do all things through him who strengthens me" (Phil. 4:13). But without Him, I am incapable of dealing with all this in my own strength and power. And I wanted to know what God's Word says about all these strong emotions I was experiencing.

In January 2023, I felt restless, not able to find the right book to help me. After talking with some friends who both had children who lived through cancer, I quickly learned that normal isn't normal anymore after cancer.

And then one day, I felt it. It was the Lord calling me to write my own book about this issue of navigating life after cancer. And here we are. This is my journey. It doesn't mean that your journey will look exactly like this. But cancer is hard no matter what the journey looks like. And life after cancer is just as hard. The emotional journey I went on wasn't something anyone told me to expect. I had to navigate it all on my own until I started voicing my concerns. Then I remembered all the wonderful friends who visited me, checked in on me, prayed for me, and sent me cards and text messages. All I had to do was cry out and share my concerns, and they would be there for me again. They were. And they still are.

This book is for anyone who has gone through this journey and isn't sure what God wants them to do with all the feelings. This book is for anyone who has watched a loved one walk this journey and isn't sure how to help them find a new normal. This book is for anyone who wants to hear what God says about recovery from a trauma that's as real as it gets.

I pray that reading about my journey will help you have a better understanding of what cancer really looks like. I pray that reading what God's Word says about the gamut of emotions you or your family members might experience will bring you comfort and encouragement to face the continuing battle. I pray that you will come to know that with God, we can do hard things; He is faithful through it all.

Your steadfast love, O LORD, extends to the heavens,
your faithfulness to the clouds.

—Ps. 36:5

Part I:

MY CANCER JOURNEY

There was no reason to be nervous. It was a routine mammogram. I'd done it dozens of times, every year like clockwork. I had always been intentional about making sure to get a yearly mammogram, not for any particular reason. It just made sense to take care of myself.

There was only one instance where I had been nervous. I'd gotten a call from the breast center telling me they needed to do an ultrasound on something they found during the mammogram. I immediately went to the worst-case scenario, but my husband, Kurt, cautioned me against thinking that way. He went with me to the ultrasound appointment for support. The radiologist looked at the imaging quickly and said it was a benign cyst. He said I could probably expect more of them as I got older. Okay. No big deal. I was able to move on.

Another time, I received a call for an ultrasound after something showed up on my routine mammogram. But I wasn't nervous this time. I just assumed it was another benign cyst.

Kurt offered to come with me, but I declined. I was certain there was no reason to worry.

I was familiar with what would happen. A technician would plop a cold, goopy, Vaseline-type substance on my breast and take multiple images with a wand-like instrument. Then she'd send the images to the radiologist who would decide the next steps. Either I could leave, or they'd refer me onward.

After the ultrasound, the technician draped a cloth over my breasts and left the room for what felt like an eternity. She finally returned and said the radiologist could not say with 100 percent certainty that this was simply a benign cyst. He recommended a biopsy be performed as soon as possible.

And in that moment, I knew. I knew instantly that I had breast cancer. I had never uttered those words, but something in my spirit told me it was cancer. I asked if the biopsy would hurt. She said it might pinch a little, but there wouldn't be much pain, especially since they numb the area before the procedure. She said they would schedule it quickly and told me not to worry. She said it was probably nothing, but I knew she was wrong.

A couple days passed before I returned to the breast center for my biopsy. This time, I was a nervous wreck. I'd never had a biopsy before. I had no idea what to expect. The nurse who would be with me throughout the process brought me to the room where the procedure would be performed. It was cold, sterile, and dimly lit. It felt as if they were trying to create some sort of romantic ambiance. There was nothing romantic about what I was feeling.

After being alone in that room with my thoughts and fears for about 20 minutes, the nurse finally returned and explained the process. She assured me that they would numb the area of the breast and that I shouldn't feel anything but a pinch. They would find the area of concern with an ultrasound before making a very small incision. There would be clicking sounds when the doctor removed the biopsy samples. It wouldn't hurt, and it shouldn't take long. She kept repeating that it wouldn't hurt, but I'm here to tell you she was wrong.

They did numb the area, but I felt everything they did, including the incision. The incision was just a pulling and stretching of the skin, but then they inserted the instruments to do the biopsy. That's what hurt. I heard a click, and then one of the instruments was removed and reinserted. There was another click, and the process was repeated three times. The pain was pretty intense, and my body was stiff from tension and fear. I was told to relax. Sure. I'll get right on that. And then it was over.

Everyone left the room so I could put my gown back on. I could feel my right breast throbbing with pain, and I was anxious to get home to take some Tylenol. The nurse returned to walk me to the dressing room and said it would be a few days before I got the results. Someone would call me as soon as they knew something.

The biopsy took place on a Thursday. By Friday, I was visibly bruised and sore. But I was also excited. I was going to our church's women's retreat for the weekend. I rode with my dear friends that afternoon. They were anxious for an update on how things went, so we talked about it on the way to our destination. A lot of people from church knew about my biopsy and were praying for me during the procedure. Many people wanted to know what happened and offered to continue to pray for the results to be negative for cancer. But I knew. I didn't tell anyone that I knew. They would certainly dismiss my "knowing" as simply being nervous. But I just knew.

The entire weekend was spent in God's Word, worshiping Him, praying to Him, and fellowshipping in amazing ways. Many women prayed for me that weekend. I felt such peace. But I still knew. It was the first glimpse of the faithfulness of God that I would come to experience over the next 10 months. In fact, the theme for that weekend was God's faithfulness. I was meant to be there.

We returned Sunday afternoon. I was happy to be home with Kurt and our fur babies, Max and Maggie. I didn't have much going on the next day with the exception of preparing to teach that week for our women's Bible study. So I put my efforts into the study that day. I was hoping for a call with the report, but it never came.

The next morning, Tuesday, March 8, 2022, there was a leaders' meeting for the women's Bible study. All the facilitators for our study met on Tuesday mornings to prepare for our time with the ladies in our groups the following day. As my fellow leaders arrived, they all wanted to know if I'd gotten any results yet. I told them no. But just as the meeting was about to begin, my phone rang. I took it into the empty sanctuary where I could take the call in private.

"Hello," I said. "This is Theresia."

The woman on the other end gave me her name, but I don't remember what it was. She had a sweet voice and was very calming, but she was straight to the point.

"I have the results of your biopsy," she said. "I'm afraid we did find cancer cells in your biopsy."

I knew.

Even though I already knew, hearing those words was surreal. I felt as if I was watching myself from the ceiling of the sanctuary. I said, "Okay. What's next?" I was ready to go. Let's get this thing out of me.

She informed me that a breast surgeon would be in touch with me very soon to talk about the next steps. Breast surgeon? Why would I need a breast surgeon? I didn't ask that question, but I did ask, "What stage is it? What kind is it?" The nice lady didn't have any specifics and said the breast surgeon would be able to explain all those details to me when we met. And with that, we ended the call.

I called my husband. He answered quickly, and I said, "I have breast cancer." I didn't cry. I told him, "I knew." He sounded shocked and concerned but said, "Okay. I'm so sorry, but just like we did with *my* cancer, we will get through this together, okay? We will see what the surgeon has to say, and we'll go from there." (Kurt had been diagnosed with Stage 3 melanoma 10 years earlier, and he came through his treatments well.) He asked if I wanted him to come home. I told him I was at the leaders' meeting and wanted to stay there. I told him I'd be home by noon. He said he would try to come home early. We said, "I love you" and hung up.

I quickly walked back to the meeting and quietly sat down. Rhoda, our study coordinator at the time, looked at me with concern. She kept nodding her head as if to give me permission to share.

The room was quiet, and with all eyes on me, I said, "I have breast cancer." And with that, I burst into tears. Rhoda immediately got up, ran over to me, and put her arms around my neck. The women to my left and right grabbed me and held me as I sobbed. Rhoda began to pray. And then all 13 women in that room—all crying as well—prayed for me. I felt this unmistakable peace come over me with each and every prayer. My sobbing ended, and I just allowed the prayers to wash over me. I realized that God hadn't allowed the phone to ring on Monday because I was alone and wouldn't have had the support of these women. Instead, He allowed me to be in the presence of these godly women who prayed for me and strengthened me. The faithfulness of God was on full display.

Rhoda asked if I wanted to leave, but I knew this was where I belonged. I needed to stay.

When I got home, I immediately called my mother. She cried. I didn't. I just shared matter of factly. She was in disbelief. No mother wants to see her child suffer from a dreadful disease such as cancer. And she knew the hell I would endure because she had watched her husband, my father, die from small cell carcinoma of the lungs 10 years earlier. She was stunned and asked why I had breast cancer since there was no history of it in our family. I explained that there doesn't have to be a history of cancer for there to be cancer. It strikes randomly. She asked what I needed, and I told her I wasn't sure. I asked her if she would tell my brother, Chris, as I didn't think I could handle telling him. I also called my mother-in-law, Arlene. I am close to her and felt I owed it to her to share this news personally. She and my mother vowed their love, support, and prayers.

I texted our small group women to let them know the news. They each texted me back to let me know they would be with me through this journey. This was the faithfulness of God. When Kurt returned home, he hugged me and held me for the longest time. But I didn't cry. I felt disconnected from myself. I also felt safe in his arms as if it were all a dream. He asked what I needed, and I asked him to let his family know. I couldn't bear it. He sent a text to his family. A text seems harsh, but it really is, at times, the easiest way to communicate to multiple people. And in our case, there were more than a dozen of them.

I slept most of the afternoon. I was exhausted and drained from crying and receiving the dreadful news.

It was a couple days before I received a phone call from Dr. Spivey's office asking me to come in to meet with her. She would be my breast surgeon and the one who would introduce me to an oncologist. Prior to our meeting, I told Kurt I didn't want chemotherapy and didn't want to lose my hair. Two days later, Kurt and I met with Dr. Spivey and my nurse navigator, Trisha. Dr. Spivey did another ultrasound to see where the cancer was located. She also did a physical exam of my right breast but noted that she felt nothing, which was good because it meant the tumor was small.

Dr. Spivey rattled off so much information that it was like drinking from a fire hose. She must have seen the look of sheer horror on my face because she slowed down a bit to ask us questions and see what she needed to repeat. I was grateful that Kurt was with me so he could ask more detailed questions. I had no idea what was happening to me. I didn't know what questions to ask. I felt as if I was there just for the ride.

Dr. Spivey explained that I had stage 1 triple-negative breast cancer (TNBC), which accounts for 10 to 20 percent of all breast cancers. It is an aggressive form of cancer and does not have estrogen or hormone receptors, making treatment difficult. It also grows and spreads more quickly than other breast cancers. She explained the course of treatment, which would include chemotherapy (I would lose my hair), a lumpectomy, and radiation. That would take place Monday through Friday for four to six weeks. I was stunned. At the same time, I was grateful for Dr. Spivey and Trisha who sat with me and Kurt long after closing time to explain the details and answer all our questions. I was grateful that the word *mastectomy* never came up in the conversation.

Next up was a breast MRI and then the placement of a SCOUT, a device that would show them where the cancer was when it was time to do the lumpectomy after chemotherapy. I would then meet with my oncologist and have a port placement. Then I would start treatment.

Kurt and I went out to dinner after our meeting with Dr. Spivey, and I asked a ton of questions about things I didn't understand. My head was spinning, but Kurt was ever so patient, kind, and caring as he explained things. I didn't get much sleep that night with all this newfound information swirling in my head.

A few days after meeting with Dr. Spivey, I had my breast MRI. Once again, I was a nervous wreck. An IV was placed, and the technician prepared me for the scan. I had to lie on my stomach as she placed each breast in a hole that they then secured. Then they moved me into the MRI machine. I was so nervous that once I laid on my stomach and got settled, I vomited on the board I was lying on. We had to start over. Eventually, I settled down and got through the MRI.

Next, the SCOUT device was implanted. It was a quick procedure that didn't hurt at all (unlike the biopsy), and I was grateful. I was told that the doctors would use a device to scan for the SCOUT when it was time for the lumpectomy. They allowed me to listen to what it sounded like and assured me I wouldn't set off alarms at security checkpoints at the airport. It was a moment of levity in a serious situation.

Finally, I had the opportunity to meet my oncologist, Dr. Janelle Miller. She, too, is a cancer survivor—of thyroid cancer. I knew she would understand my fear and angst. She was such a calming presence. Kurt and I both instantly liked her, just as we did Dr. Spivey. Dr. Miller spent about two hours with us explaining the various facets of what I would face while going through chemotherapy. I would have eight cycles, or rounds, one every two weeks for a total of four months. She told me I'd be on three types of chemotherapy medicines: Adriamycin—also known as the "red devil"—Cytoxan, and AC-Taxol (AC-T). The first two, Adriamycin and Cytoxan, would be given to me during the first four cycles, and Taxol would be given to me during the last four cycles. Adriamycin causes your hair to fall out. The chemotherapy drugs would be accompanied by a litany of other drugs to help with side effects, keep my blood counts in normal ranges, and combat reactions, if any.

I asked Dr. Miller if I would vomit a lot. I hate vomiting. It makes me vomit. She explained that most chemotherapy drugs don't make you vomit like in years past. Vomiting is possible, but it's not severe. Chemo does make you nauseous, but they would give me medicines to combat that.

I would have my blood drawn through a port in my chest before each cycle could begin to make sure all my lab counts were in the normal range. Anything out of the norm would mean I couldn't have chemotherapy that week. I prayed that this would never be the case because I wanted this to be over before it even started.

The first two drugs would take about four hours to administer. The Taxol would take about six hours. I knew it would be a long summer. I was ready to get started. The sooner I started, the sooner I could get it over with and be cancer-free.

But first I had to have an echocardiogram to make sure my heart was strong enough to withstand the effects of the Adriamycin and Cytoxan—yet another appointment. I was astonished at how many scans and tests I had to have before I could even start my treatments.

By this point, our women's Bible study was over for the season, so I was grateful I could simply spend my days concentrating on doctors' appointments. I went to the echocardiogram alone. I'd had one before, so again, I wasn't worried. I knew I had tachycardia and worried it might make my heart not strong enough for the chemo drugs. The technician started an IV to do contrast dye and was well into the process of doing the ECG when the lights went out and the machine shut down. The entire building had a power outage. Everyone was worried that the information retrieved from the ECG to that point hadn't been saved yet, and if it wasn't saved, I'd have to come back another day to do it all over again. Thankfully, the information had saved, and all was well. The results pointed to my heart being strong enough for chemo. I was grateful. It was one less thing to worry about. There would be enough side effects to deal with. I didn't need to worry about my heart as well.

I also had to have a PET scan to ensure that the cancer hadn't spread and to get a baseline for my current situation. I had to wait an hour to let what they injected into my veins make its way throughout my body before they could perform the scan. As I waited, I opened the Bible app on my phone. It literally opened to Jeremiah 17:14: "Heal me, O Lord, and I shall be healed; save me, and I shall be saved, for you are my praise." A gentle peace settled over me while I waited, and I knew I would be okay during this scan too.

Dr. Miller's office was finally able to get my port placement scheduled for March 30. If all went well, I would start chemo on March 31. Kurt and I decided to take a long weekend prior to everything starting, and we set our sights on getting away. We wanted to have a special time of togetherness without thinking about the things that were in our immediate future. We left on a Thursday for a wonderful long weekend away. It was just what I needed—to concentrate and focus on just us, to be honest about the journey we were about to embark on, and to rest from the chaos of the last several weeks.

Ports are often used for chemotherapy patients because it saves the patient from being constantly stuck with needles due to blood draws, IV placements, and other pokes and needles. Port placement took place on Wednesday morning. It was a quick surgical procedure, but my upper left chest protruded with this new device that would be my constant companion for nine months until it was removed.

My chest was sore that evening and the next day when I reported for my first day of chemotherapy. Because of COVID-19 restrictions and other concerns for the health and well-being of other patients, I had to wear a mask when I was in the oncology offices, especially the infusion room.

I had no idea what to expect, and once more, I was incredibly nervous. In fact, I was quite terrified. All chemo patients had to have someone with them during their treatment and available to drive them home. Kurt received permission from work to attend chemo sessions with me for the duration. He got extra time off as a caregiver so he wouldn't have to use sick days or vacation hours. We knew we'd be in the infusion room for several hours, so we stopped to pick up something to snack on once when we got settled. We both ordered something sweet. We felt like we deserved it.

We arrived, got checked in, and settled into the waiting room, which was filled with hematology and cancer patients. By this point, I was scared to death. Finally, a nurse called my name, and Kurt and I went with her into the infusion room. Nurses were bustling around the room, caring for the patients in chairs that were to my right. There were four rows, each with four large, comfy-looking, recliner-type chairs. Next to them were smaller, less comfortable chairs. Abbie introduced herself and said she'd be taking care of me. She was so sweet and kind, but all I could focus on were the people in the large chairs. There were so many of them. I looked around the room, and all I could think was that "I am one of them now. I am a cancer patient." I wanted to run from the room and burst into tears. Abbie touched my arm and suggested I sit in one of the chairs. Kurt sat next to me in the less comfortable chair.

Abbie explained that she would draw my labs first to make sure we could start chemo. The area of my port was incredibly sore, so drawing for blood was painful, but she explained that it was because my port had been placed just a day earlier. It normally isn't painful. Abbie wasn't able to get any blood out of my port. She tried and tried but was unsuccessful. That meant there might be a clog in the port, so she had to give me heparin, a blood thinner, to unclog it. That meant we would have to wait 20 to 30 minutes to let the medicine do its thing before she could try to draw blood again. So we sat and waited, and snacked on our yummy treats.

While we waited, I watched everything that was going on in the infusion room. It was a room filled with genuinely caring nurses looking after each person attentively and specifically. They rushed but not in a way that was alarming. They just had work that needed to be done. Abbie was among them. She checked in on me every so often. "You okay?" she'd ask. Outside of being nervous, I was fine. I think she knew I was a nervous wreck, and it was a comfort to have her ask.

She eventually returned to try to draw blood. The port still wouldn't cooperate. She gave me another round of heparin, and we waited another 20 to 30 minutes. After a third round of heparin and another wait, she finally got blood to come out. Hallelujah! But the lab now had to check the blood. That meant another wait of 15 minutes or so. Abbie returned and said the labs were normal. We could commence with chemotherapy.

"Okay," I thought. "Here we go."

I was told to take my oral anti-nausea medicine. They started me on a drip of a steroid to combat nausea and any chance of a negative reaction. That took about 30 minutes. Abbie returned when it was finished and asked what flavor I wanted.

"What?" I asked, stupefied.

She said it was time for the Adriamycin, which can cause mouth sores. Munching on ice chips or flavored popsicles help combat the mouth sores. I chose grape. Abbie told me she'd be right back with the two chemo drugs.

When Abbie returned, I nearly fell out of my chair. Prior to leaving, she had been wearing everyday scrubs and a mask. Now she was covered from head to toe in hazmat-like gear. She wore a white gown that covered her entire body and was tied in the back. She wore a mask and a face shield that covered her entire face. She had on gloves that went over her white gown and all the way up to her elbows. In her hands was an IV bag of Cytoxan and two huge syringes filled with some type of red liquid. That was the red devil.

I remember thinking to myself, "What in the world is she about to put into my body that she needs to protect herself in such a manner?" Suddenly I was petrified. I prayed to God to protect me from harm.

Abbie showed me the syringes of Adriamycin. It's what they call a "push drug." They push the medicine into the body through the port instead of using an IV drip bag. That process didn't take very long. Then she connected me to the bag of Cytoxan, which took about two hours to administer.

While the chemo drugs were being administered, I tried to read the Psalms but found my mind wandering. I kept looking at the people in the other chairs. I wondered what type of cancer they had. How long had they had it? Had it spread? Which one of us would die first from this disease called cancer? One woman slept the entire time I was there, and it was clear that she had already been there a few hours prior to my arrival. She wore a wig and looked weak but pretty. She even wore makeup. I wanted to strike up a conversation with her and pray for her, but she slept on.

Kurt and I finished our sweet snacks and tried laughing about things, but it seemed empty. While we visited with one another, one man was able to ring the bell. His family had come and brought him balloons to celebrate the end of his chemo. I couldn't see everything that happened because my back was to them, but I knew that every nurse stopped what they were doing and gathered around as the man read a few lines from the inscription on the bell. One of the nurses videotaped the entire event. When he rang the bell three times, the entire room erupted in cheers and applause. For the first time since my diagnosis, I cried. I cried for joy for the man, and I cried in sadness for me because my bell-ringing time was still so far from reality.

Abbie came over to me and said, "This is your first one. But soon enough, you'll be ringing the bell too. Look forward to that, and let that keep you going." Her words were such a comfort, and I appreciated her effort to encourage me.

Finally, my drip bag was empty, and my machine beeped incessantly. Abbie came over and said, "Well, that was cycle one. You're all done. You can check out and go home."

I couldn't believe it. I was finished. Only seven more to go. And I felt fine—so far. I almost felt like celebrating, but I also wondered how long it would be before I began to feel the effects of the chemo drugs.

Intense fatigue started about a day after that first treatment. I had a little back pain and flushing in my face, and the nausea kicked in as well. I became winded trying to walk up the stairs in my house. The best I could do was lie on the couch and sleep—a lot. I had been told to rest a lot for three days after the chemo, and I was more than happy to oblige. Thankfully, I had anti-nausea medicine and never vomited. The fatigue, however, got worse with each and every cycle of treatment.

A sweet friend from church who had previously had the same type of breast cancer told me of her experience with AC-T. She explained that she was able to walk a mile or so nearly every day while going through chemo and that the exercise was critical in her healing process. I couldn't walk to the mailbox in front of my house without feeling winded and completely exhausted. And this was worse than just being exhausted. I felt that every ounce of strength in my body had been sucked out of me and replaced with chemotherapy drugs. I quickly learned that not everyone responds to chemo the same. And my journey would be vastly different than my friend's.

I started a CaringBridge journal for those who wanted to keep track of my progress and pray for me. CaringBridge is an online diary that can be updated as often as the person wants. I ultimately shared it with everyone in my church. I knew that many people in my church body were praying for me, and I was so grateful for all of them.

CaringBridge Journal Update, April 4, 2022: I hate to share all of this as I fear it sounds as if I'm complaining. I'm really not. I know that despite all of these terrible feelings, God is working a miracle inside my body. I just can't see it. But I know the chemo is doing all that it's supposed to do to make me healthy once again. We are trusting in the One who is in control over all of what's happening inside my body.

The evening prior to starting chemo, we received the first of many meals that would be delivered. Friends and church people delivered meals every Monday, Wednesday, and Friday for the entire time I went through chemotherapy. It was such a gift and a blessing to us so we could simply focus on my health care and well-being. Each meal was simply amazing.

My mother came to Indianapolis where we lived about a week after my first chemo and stayed for 16 days. We were grateful for her help since we didn't know how chemo would impact me. She quickly got into a rhythm of coming to Indianapolis for every chemo treatment. Kurt went to the treatments with me (my mother came with me to two appointments), and then my mother did an amazing job of caring for me. While I was lying on the couch feeling incredible fatigue and pain, she brought me Tylenol, cleaned my house, and brought meals to me. She helped me up the stairs when I was too weak to walk and took care of our animals every day. She stayed each time for five to seven days and then went home only to come back again two weeks later. She was such an incredible help to me and Kurt.

About a week after my first chemo treatment, I began having intense muscle spasms in my lower back. Every time I moved, I had a spasm. It didn't matter if I was standing, sitting, or lying down, I'd have spasms that lasted about a full minute.

The pain was unreal. Dr. Miller explained that it was probably the bone marrow in my back working overtime to increase my white blood cell counts. She mentioned that since I experienced muscle spasms after the first cycle, I would likely have them after each treatment. It was something to look forward to, I guess.

I was also expecting to start seeing my hair fall out, which I was not looking forward to. I decided not to shave my head. I felt that cancer was already taking so much from me that I wasn't going to allow it to force me to shave my head. I wanted to keep as much hair as possible for as long as possible. Call me stubborn, I guess, but my hair is important to me. It's part of what makes me who I am. I bought hats—lots of hats—for when I did start losing my hair. I promised everyone that if I was going to be bald, I was going to be stylish and cute.

It was finally time for cycle two of chemotherapy. We had the same issues with the port as we had the first time. That meant a much longer stay in the infusion room than the four hours I was expecting. My mother was able to go to this treatment with me, and it was such a comfort to have her there. Once again, I tried sleeping or reading the Psalms during the steroid and chemo drips, but I was too consumed with watching what was happening to other people. I kept wondering what they were going through, how they were responding to this dreadful disease, and if they knew the God who saves and heals. I wanted desperately to tell everyone about Him, but I resisted, mostly because those closest to me were asleep.

Thankfully, my taste buds never changed, and I was able to fully enjoy all the wonderful meals people provided for us. But the nausea was as real as it gets. After this second round of chemo, I required anti-nausea medicine. But again, I never vomited. I did have some new side effects, however. I didn't have mouth sores but rather nose sores. Even Abbie said this was rather odd, and they gave me a prescription for some ointment. I was also suffering with extremely dry mouth. Lifesavers were a life saver!

CaringBridge Journal Update, April 18, 2022: I've started losing my hair. It started the day I had chemo. At first it was slowly coming out, but now it's coming out by the handful. To be very honest, I'm not dealing with it well. I can't articulate why. I just feel like I'm losing a part of myself. Some people say, "It's only hair." But it's more than that to me. I know God has a purpose and a plan even in the hair loss.

I had intense muscle spasms again, and the intensity increased with each chemo cycle. And this time, the fatigue was incredibly intense. I couldn't believe that a person could sleep so much yet still be so exhausted. But this was my new normal.

Many people continually asked how they could help. I honestly didn't know what to tell them. I had everything I needed. We had meals lined up for the next four months. My mother was cleaning the house when she was with us. The dog and cat were well cared for. I didn't have any other specific tangible needs that needed to be addressed. I prayed about how people could help me, and the only thing the Lord showed me that I needed was companionship. I am such a people person, and I usually kept a very busy schedule of meeting with people and being involved in ministry.

I had to back away from several ministries I was involved in at church, including the writing team that was preparing for our next women's Bible study. I had also missed several monthly missions team meetings. I was, however, able to still write the missions team monthly newsletter. Our weekly women's Bible study was now over, and I missed the ladies in my group. Lunches with friends were few and far between. I was very lonely during my chemotherapy. I missed my tribe—my people. I was receiving dozens of cards each week, but I needed physical presence. So I told everyone to come and visit me. People began to schedule time to visit on the days I felt best, which was usually the week I didn't have chemo. I slept most of the time on the days following chemo, so I usually had no visitors during that time. Before I knew it, I had so many people signed up to visit me that my entire calendar was filled for four months. What a blessing to me! It truly was life-giving to have so many women come and spend an hour or two visiting with me. The conversations were joy-filled, and they invigorated me. Of course, I slept a few hours after they left, but I still felt so alive.

CaringBridge Journal Update, April 29, 2022: I must confess, chemotherapy is dragging on incredibly slow. I'm trying desperately to live life as normally as I can, but the fatigue is exhausting. Pun intended. And I feel as if I live for the end of all of this. I want my old life back, but that isn't going to happen. I will never return to where I was before, and finding acceptance in that has been hard on this journey.

I would have about three to four fairly good days between the fatigue and the muscle spasms in my back. I tried to enjoy those good days as best as I could. But the fatigue was overwhelming, even on the good days.

My oncologist had encouraged me to have genetic testing to see if there were indicators that my cancer might return. It was a simple blood test that would be able to tell us so much more about the cancer that was now inside of me. A few days after my last chemo treatment, I received the results of my genetic testing. It showed a positive result for a genetic mutation, BARD1, which indicates that there might be a recurrence of the cancer. This particular mutation causes the type of cancer I already have, so it made sense that it could recur. The challenge is that this mutation is a relatively new one, and there aren't a lot of statistics or data on it.

In other words, there isn't enough information to tell me I have a 90 percent chance of it recurring or a 5 percent chance of it coming back. There also isn't enough data to help provide supporting guidance on what type of action I should take. Do I get a mastectomy or not? We didn't really know enough to make an informed decision yet. Kurt and I scheduled a meeting with a genetic counselor, but it would be unlikely that she would be able to provide us with more information to make that decision.

The visit with the genetic counselor was overwhelming. There was so much information that I felt exhausted when it was over. She shared that women have about a 12 percent chance of getting breast cancer in their lifetime. Because of the particular genetic mutation I have, I had a 15 to 40 percent chance of developing breast cancer. Now that breast cancer was a reality, the risk of recurrence for me had increased. However, because the variant is so new, they didn't have enough data to tell me what that percentage of recurrence might be. So they couldn't say for certain that it would come back at fill-in-the-blank percent. She also noted that the type of mutation doesn't have enough information on it to call for a bilateral (or double) mastectomy as some others would suggest. That meant I had no more information than I had before I walked in the door as to whether or not I should have a bilateral mastectomy.

If I opted to keep my breasts, the course of care for the rest of my life would include a mammogram and then an MRI six months later, and then in another six months, a mammogram, and back and forth forever. What I needed to decide was whether or not I could handle the anxiety that would come with these scans every six months. Also, could I handle having a recurrence of cancer and going through chemotherapy again? These were the questions I needed to answer for myself, and they would guide me in making a decision on whether or not to keep my breasts.

The other questions were about surgery. We knew the risks of not having surgery, but what were the risks of having surgery? Thankfully, I didn't have to make a decision right at that moment. I had five more cycles of chemotherapy left, and I could wait until the very last one to make that decision.

CaringBridge Journal Update, May 9, 2022:
Everywhere I turn lately, the same scripture verse keeps popping up. It has become such a great comfort to me, reminding me every time I see it that God is at work,

and I can rest in His promises. "Do not fear, for I am with you. Do not be dismayed, for I am your God, I will strengthen you, I will help you. I will uphold you with my righteous right hand" (Isa. 41:10).

I was finally at the halfway point of chemo, and the port worked the very first time in an attempt to draw blood for labs. It usually took some calisthenics and heparin or alteplase to get the blood to flow, but this time it worked like a charm. I was thrilled. Unfortunately, I immediately felt crummy after the chemo, and it stuck around for quite a while. But for now, I could rejoice in knowing that Adriamycin and Cytoxan were in my past. I was preparing for Taxol that, I was promised, would be much kinder to me.

Kurt and I met with Dr. Spivey, my breast surgeon, on May 23 for an exam and another ultrasound. She literally gasped and shouted with joy. My tumor was now microscopic in size. All I could do was rejoice in how God was working through modern medicine to kill the tumor.

Dr. Spivey also talked in depth with us about my options for surgery. She was very forthcoming about many details, including ones I didn't really want to know about. She also shared what I would experience during and after reconstruction surgery and how each surgery would affect me. Having the bilateral mastectomy would reduce my chance of the cancer returning by 95 to 97 percent. Those are pretty good odds. She encouraged us to meet with her partner, Dr. Sando, who would do the reconstructive surgery. They wanted me to make a decision soon since they wanted to schedule surgery for three to five weeks after my last chemo. Since mine is a fast-growing cancer, they didn't want to take any chances that something lingering would start to grow. Dr. Spivey assured me she wasn't going to pressure me one way or the other and that it was totally my decision.

My introduction to Taxol at round five of chemotherapy wasn't a good one. I was in the infusion room far longer than I had expected. Part of it was that they couldn't get the port to cooperate for labs again, and they spent nearly two hours on that alone. Once it finally worked, I started with pre-meds of Pepcid, more steroids, and Benadryl before they started the Taxol. Thankfully, I didn't have any type of reaction as is common with Taxol. The Benadryl made me incredibly tired, but there was so much activity in the infusion room that I wasn't able to sleep. I drifted in and out but couldn't sleep the way I wanted to. I did get a good nap once I got home, and I didn't feel too bad that first day.

I woke up the next day in excruciating pain all over my body. Taxol had not been kind to me as everyone had promised. I was so grateful that my mother was there. She and Kurt had to do everything except bathe me because I was in too much pain to do it on my own. Walking was very painful, and all I could do was lie on the couch and moan in pain. I was able to get in touch with someone from the oncology office. They suggested extra strength Tylenol alternating with ibuprofen. They said that if the pain was this bad again, they might have to put me on a narcotic. I was dreading the thought. They also recommended Icy Hot, which helped a little. All I could do was dread the next three cycles.

Somewhere in the middle of all the pain, I ended up having an allergic reaction to something. I had hives and itched all over. I took tramadol and Benadryl, both of which helped.

In cycle six of chemotherapy, they increased my steroids to help alleviate the pain I'd been experiencing. While I was there, I was able to meet with a nurse practitioner who determined that I was probably allergic to Taxol. She said I should take prednisone for four days following each round of chemo. And I was to take tramadol the Friday night after chemo. I needed a road map just to keep up with all the medicines I had to take at home. My medicine cabinet began to look like a mini-pharmacy. By Saturday night and Sunday morning, the pain was incredibly intense despite taking tramadol. I was encouraged to take extra strength Tylenol on top of the tramadol. It helped and allowed me to have a restful sleep for a few hours. I knew this is what I had to look forward to for the last two treatments. I was dreading it, but at the same time I was grateful I didn't have another allergic reaction.

Between treatments, Kurt and I met with Dr. Sando. He did a wonderful job of giving us a lot of things to consider and answered many of our questions. We both left feeling that God had surrounded us with the best in care from every perspective and position.

CaringBridge Journal Update, June 24, 2022: I really struggled with this for several days. It's one thing to have a doctor tell you that it's absolutely necessary to have a mastectomy for your health. However, I have not received those words from any of my doctors. It is a decision that I have to make based on what is going to be best for me emotionally, psychologically, and spiritually. Yet I feel this is entirely unnatural to ask any woman to make such a decision. And it's not easy at all. I have decided, however, to move forward with having the bilateral mastectomy. It's been hell, and I can't go through this again. I also know there is a lot of risk to my body to have to have chemo again. That was the biggest reason for making this decision. If I can prevent the cancer from coming back, I'll do it. It won't be easy, but it will be temporary. Surgery is scheduled for August 15 followed by the implant surgery a few months after that.

July 7, 2022, was my last chemotherapy treatment. Abbie was the nurse who cared for me the first day of chemotherapy, and she was there for me on my last day of chemotherapy. It was so meaningful to me. She said, "I was with you in the beginning, and I wanted to see you through to the end." She also reminded me of my reaction the first time I walked into the infusion room.

"Your eyes were as big as saucers," she said. "You were terrified. But you got through it. And in a few hours, you're going to ring that bell. I'm so proud of you."

My mom was with me for this treatment that lasted five hours, thanks to yet a still cantankerous port. When it was over, Kurt and his mom, Arlene, joined us in the infusion room. Arlene gave me a beautiful breast cancer bracelet to celebrate my victory. She and my mom, as well as Kurt, had been there for me through it all, and I wanted all of them there on my last day.

When I was finished, Abbie took me over to the bell, and everyone stopped what they were doing, including the nurses. They gathered around me as I uttered (barely) the words inscribed on the bell. I rang the bell three times and threw my hands in the air in victory. The room erupted in applause. I will never forget the hug from my husband. All the nurses hugged me as did my mom and Arlene. That moment will forever be etched in my mind.

The four of us were going to go out to eat and celebrate. After checkout, we headed outside. As we exited the elevator, I saw someone who looked familiar. I looked more and then saw someone else I knew. When I walked out the front door, every woman from my small group, the women in my summer Bible study, and most of Kurt's family were standing in a semi-circle. They had balloons, flowers, and posters, and they were ringing bells in my honor. They were all there to celebrate with me the victory that was now mine. I will forever cherish that memory.

After hugs to each and every person, someone started praying, and others joined in. Then someone spontaneously started singing the beautiful hymn "Great Is Thy Faithfulness." I sobbed because no one knew that this was my favorite hymn and that I had indeed seen the faithfulness of God through the last four months since my diagnosis.

We eventually said goodbye to our friends, and the rest of the family was able to join us for an early dinner celebration. Every one of those people had carried me through this difficult journey, and they were there to celebrate with me in the end.

CaringBridge Journal Update, July 8, 2022: This is what it looks like to kick cancer's butt! Get on your knees and pray. Trust the Lord to carry you through and to be faithful. Surround yourself with family, friends, and a body of believers who will pray for you and feed you and care for you and cry with you and celebrate with you. Keep getting on your knees to pray. And don't forget the faithfulness of God. And He is truly a faithful God.

The days following that last chemo treatment were filled with tears of joy and lots of pain. I moaned a lot, but I also smiled a lot. All around me, I had the posters, balloons, and flowers from my friends and family. I realized in those dark days of pain that with God, we can do hard things.

Prior to my cancer diagnosis, we had planned to move my mother in with us. Then cancer came calling. Now that chemo was over, we were finally able to get her moved in. She wanted to be in our home before my mastectomy surgery so she could be there to help me during recovery. While we waited for the surgery, she flew home for a week or so to pack up as much as she could. On July 27, I flew down to her home to help her.

Prior to my departure to South Carolina, I had a lot of post-chemo imaging, including an MRI, a mammogram, and an ultrasound. We also met with my breast surgeon, Dr. Spivey, who said all the imaging showed good response. In fact, there was no evidence of the tumor (or any other tumors at all). God is faithful!

On my travels south, I was in a wheelchair at the airports since I didn't have the strength to walk to the gates on my own.

I was in South Carolina for nearly three weeks. Kurt drove down and loaded up our SUV before taking some things back home to Indiana. The movers came and loaded up my mom's belongings. A couple days later, we packed up my mom's SUV and said a tearful goodbye to my childhood home. It was a tough goodbye for both of us, especially since it had been her home for nearly 40 years.

I slept a lot while I was at my mother's home. My strength and energy were zapped, but I do feel I provided some emotional support for her. At least that's my hope. We drove up to Indianapolis on August 11. We unloaded her car and got her as settled as possible. Thankfully, her furniture wouldn't be delivered for three weeks, so we didn't have to worry about that for the time being. Once we were back in Indianapolis, we spent the weekend preparing for my surgery on Monday morning.

I was noticing a little more energy, but I was far from being back to normal. I tired easily and still required a daily nap, which was just fine with me. I was told it would be four to six weeks before the chemo was out of my body, but it could take up to a year before I felt back to normal.

CaringBridge Journal Update, July 14, 2023: I have been struggling mightily leading up to tomorrow's surgery. The last three weeks had me ruminating throughout the day and having nightmares at night. Sleep has been hard to come by, so I am actually looking forward to uninterrupted sleep for 5 to 6 hours tomorrow. However, I know that it was no coincidence that I was at church this morning to hear

"Battle Belongs" (Phil Wickham), which has been my anthem throughout this journey. And then to hear (pastor) Drew's message on the comfort our Heavenly Father brings to those who are suffering. I look forward to the day when I am able to comfort someone else in the way I have received so much comfort from both our Lord and from others within the Body of Christ.

Sleep didn't come easily for me the night before surgery. I felt such intense grief, and I was flooded with emotion although I was able to stifle it. Our 5:00 a.m. arrival time came early, and the streets were empty as we drove to Women's Hospital. We didn't wait long before they called us back and prepped me for surgery. My mom and Kurt were finally able to be with me. A nurse popped in every once in a while to check on me, but mostly we were alone for a while. Before I knew it, I began to sob. My husband held me as I cried uncontrollably. I was inconsolable as I realized that I was losing my breasts and nothing would make me normal again—not even new boobs. I tried to compose myself as Kurt encouraged me to feel what I was feeling.

Eventually I settled down, and Dr. Spivey came in to see me. She could tell I had been crying and quickly hugged me, all the while assuring me that I would be okay. She explained how she would cut through the center of my breasts, peel the skin back like a banana, and then remove the breast tissue. In this process, I would lose my nipples and the areola. I wasn't crazy about that either, but I had to deal with it. This was my reality now. She said Dr. Sando would be in to explain the remainder of the surgical process, including my tissue expanders.

When Dr. Sando arrived, I was mostly composed again, and he drew marks on my chest. He explained that he would place the tissue expanders once the breast tissue was removed, and that these expanders would make way for my implants. I had opted to go smaller in my reconstruction than the triple D's I was going into surgery with. I wasn't entirely sure what to expect with the tissue expanders, but I would soon find out. All I knew is that I was emotionally drained and ready for a nap.

The anesthesiologist arrived and gave me some pre-meds that made me sleepy. I don't even remember saying goodbye to my family or being wheeled out of the room into the operating room. I vaguely remember being awakened in a hospital room when Kurt and my mother walked in. They were so excited and relieved to see me, and I was glad to see them. A nurse was with me, and she explained that all went well with the surgery.

The nurse tried to get me situated and comfortable as I was trying to greet Kurt and my mom. Because of continuing COVID-19 restrictions, I was only allowed two visitors. I was actually quite okay with that now that I was in my room. I was too tired and too nauseous to receive anyone else.

Before I knew it, I started vomiting—a lot. The nurse said it was probably a reaction to the anesthesia, which I found strange since I'd never had a reaction before. It lasted about an hour, and then I felt a bit more comfortable. Two hours later, I was eating a light meal of scrambled eggs and toast. Thankfully, I was able to keep it down. I had absolutely no pain and was feeling pretty good, which surprised me. But I knew the good feelings wouldn't last long.

My mom and Kurt stayed a few hours before saying goodnight. I was ready for some sleep, although I knew it would be interrupted by nurses quite regularly. I was surprised at how often I had to use the restroom. I couldn't get out of bed by myself, so I was constantly ringing a nurse for help. A nurse also came in from time to time to drain the tubes that were sticking out of my sides. Again, I had absolutely no pain, and I enjoyed it while it lasted. I slept well and was kept very comfortable while I was awake. The nursing staff at the hospital were all terrific.

The next morning, my mom and Kurt came to take me home. Again, I was still feeling no pain. Dr. Sando came in to check my incisions and drain tubes and sign off on my being released. He was quite pleased with the results of the surgery. He reminded me to take pain medicine as instructed and not wait until the pain was unbearable. I ate some breakfast—more scrambled eggs and toast—and waited for the final paperwork.

My mother helped me dress while Kurt retrieved the car. I looked down at my wounded chest but couldn't really tell what it looked like. I needed a mirror but was in no hurry to see the wounds. Now that the anesthesia was wearing off, I could feel the tissue expanders in my chest, but it still didn't hurt. I had a mastectomy pillow to place over my chest underneath the seatbelt. I was quite wobbly, but I was so grateful to see the beautiful sunshine that morning.

Maggie, our cat, and Max, our dog, were so happy to see me. Thankfully, Max didn't try to jump up on me. My mom had already put a sheet on the couch with my pillow from the bed and a blanket so I could spend time downstairs with them instead of being off by myself in the upstairs bedroom. I was grateful. I slept quite a bit, and the afternoon flew by. Before I knew it, our meal for the day had arrived. Even though my mom was there, our friends still insisted on providing meals for all of us. We would receive a few more before mom took over the cooking duties. I was hungry and ready to eat, still feeling no pain. With more pain medicine later that evening, I was in my bed by 8:00 p.m. I can't remember if I slept well, but I imagine I did, thanks to the pain meds. The next morning, I was down on the couch again with the help of my mother. Kurt was able to work from home and was in the basement where he had spent his days working during COVID. It was so good to have him home even if he wasn't at my bedside the entire day. Just knowing he was there gave me comfort and peace.

I needed help sitting up from the couch and getting off the couch. I also needed help sitting back on the couch and lying down again. At some point in the morning, I needed to use the restroom. My mom was quick to come to my aid. As I tried to sit up, I felt such intense pain in my chest that I screamed—literally screamed. I had my mastectomy pillow close to my chest, but it didn't alleviate the pain I was feeling as I moved my body from one position to the next. Standing up was incredibly painful as well. I was moaning. That's all I could muster. Sitting on the toilet wasn't quite as bad, but it sure didn't feel great either. Coming back to the couch to sit down and then lie down made me scream more. Kurt was alarmed and came upstairs. I felt as if someone was ripping my chest in two. It was the worst pain I had ever felt.

I called my breast surgeon's office. They recommended that I call the plastic surgeon's office. I was told that the tissue expanders were sutured to the muscles of the chest wall to keep them in place. The sutures would eventually dissolve, and the expanders might move some, but the pain would eventually go away. It took five days for this to happen. Every time I moved from one position to another, all I could do in response to the pain was scream. Even the pain medicines didn't help.

Every day that passed, my mother or Kurt drained my tubes. We had to measure the amount of fluid collected each day. They were careful not to cause me anymore pain. It didn't hurt; it was just uncomfortable. Kurt and my mom both handled it like it was nothing. I became frustrated that I wasn't draining fast enough. I was ready for these dangling tubes to be gone.

About three or four days after surgery, I was finally ready to take a shower and see what I looked like. I asked Kurt to help me with the shower. He walked me upstairs and started the water running to warm it up. I unbuttoned my oversized shirt and opened it.

"Oh, it doesn't look that bad," I said as I looked in the mirror.

"No, it really doesn't," Kurt said in agreement.

Then something caught my attention.

"What is that?" I screamed in horror.

I saw on my sides and underneath my armpits something that looked like huge clumps of skin. It was hideous, and I thought I would run out of the room screaming.

Kurt reminded me that at some point Dr. Sando had explained that I had a lot of excess skin after removing my breast tissue. Making the breasts smaller meant more skin that would eventually need to be removed. I had no recollection of this conversation, nor was I prepared for what I was staring at.

"It's hideous," I cried. "I'm hideous!"

I didn't want Kurt to comfort me in a hug because I knew it would be painful. But he comforted me with his words.

"It's only temporary," he reminded me. "And you're not hideous. You're still beautiful to me."

I appreciated his attempt, but I didn't believe him. Kurt helped me with my shower, but I was so ashamed of the body he was looking at. He didn't flinch once, but I believed I looked like a monster.

A week after my surgery, Dr. Spivey called to tell me the pathology report on the lymph nodes that were removed during the mastectomy. The breast tissue showed no signs of cancer. There was no evidence of disease. I was cancer-free! I shouted with joy and shared the news with my mom and Kurt before spreading the news on my CaringBridge Journal, with my small group and the rest of the family. I was told that the odds of my cancer returning were slim. That was what I wanted and needed to hear.

A few days later, I went for a post-op visit with Dr. Sando. He was pleased with the incision site healing, although he was sad to hear that I had been in so much pain. By this point, I was beyond that. I did ask him what these things under my arms were all about.

"Those are angel wings," he said, jokingly.

I replied, "If I'm going to be an angel, I'd rather have a halo."

He laughed, but I was serious. He explained the same thing Kurt had shared with me the first time I saw them and reminded me that the extra skin would be removed when I had my reconstruction surgery, whenever that would be.

Dr. Sando was ready to fill the tissue expanders with the first dose of saline to expand the skin to prepare for my implants. He had a huge syringe filled with saline, and then he inserted the needle into the center of what was now my breast. He slowly pushed the syringe. As I looked down to watch what he was doing, I could see the tissue expander slowly getting larger, increasing what was now my breast. I was shocked. Even Kurt could see it getting bigger. It was the strangest thing to see, but I didn't feel a thing. I would have the expanders filled once more in the next week, and then I'd wait for the reconstruction surgery that would hopefully be in about two months.

I had the surgery, and about three weeks later, Kurt and I celebrated our 18th wedding anniversary. He wanted to take me out to a wonderful dinner, so I got out of my mastectomy robe, had him help me with a shower again, put on my nicest oversized shirt and some capris, and off we went to dinner. As we stood at the entrance of the restaurant waiting to be taken to our table, I felt Kurt put his arm around me. He rubbed my back and then leaned over to whisper in my ear.

"How does it feel walking around without a bra on?" he asked.

"Well, thanks for reminding me that I'm not wearing one," I said. "I had forgotten about it until you reminded me." We both laughed.

It was my first time not wearing a bra since my surgery, but it would not be my last. The only thing I hated about that night were the drain tubes that accompanied us on our date. Dr. Sando wasn't quite ready to remove them. Hopefully, that would happen the following week.

Our dinner was quite romantic, and we ate to our fill. It was a time for us to reflect on all I had been through that year and the faithfulness of God. We were so grateful that we got the chance to celebrate another year of marriage. And thanks to my chemotherapy and surgery, we hoped we'd have many more to celebrate together.

The following week, Kurt went with me to Dr. Sando's office. He was pleased with the numbers that showed my output in the drain tubes was low enough that they could finally be removed. I was quite nervous and wondered if it would be painful. I had decided that nothing would be as painful as that first week after my surgery, so I assured myself I could handle it. But honestly, it was a breeze. Dr. Sando pulled, I breathed, and the tubes were out. He didn't even have to suture the holes that were left behind. They were small enough that they would close up on their own. I felt as if I could do a dance. I felt so free having those things out of me.

I had one last visit with Dr. Spivey. I had learned right before my surgery that I was her last patient. She was moving on to another office, and eventually someone else in the office would be seeing me. She was kind enough to do the post-op visit, and she, too, was pleased with the results. I was so grateful for her. She was so kind and compassionate with me when we first met and all throughout our journey together. She surrounded me with the best medical team I could ever have. I would miss her, but I was confident in her office staff to carry me through the rest of this journey.

In October, I went back to see my oncologist, Dr. Miller, for my three-month checkup. It was then that I realized that although I was cancer-free, my journey was not yet over. I would probably be doing these types of checkups for the foreseeable future, if not for the rest of my life. I didn't realize then how much that would end up bothering me. I wanted to move on with life. But my doctors had other plans.

Dr. Miller was also pleased with how my surgery turned out, and she was thrilled to know my cancer was gone. My iron levels were low, so she started me on some iron tablets designed to help my energy levels.

At some point in the process of carrying around the tissue expanders, the sutures did indeed dissolve, and one of my expanders traveled quite a distance from its original spot and was now nearly on my side. I actually felt it when it happened. I rushed to the bathroom and stared in disbelief at what I was looking at in the mirror. I was lopsided. I showed my mom, who suggested I put on an old bra, which actually helped me not look so lopsided anymore. I alerted Dr. Sando's office, and they said this was common and would eventually happen to the other expander too. We scheduled my reconstruction surgery, which would not take place for another two months. I was incredibly disappointed as I was ready to get this part over with too.

About three weeks later, my other tissue expander decided to journey from its original location to my side as well. I still had a month and a half before surgery. The lopsided tissue expanders were making my breasts look lopsided, and I still had the "angel wings." My reconstructive surgery on December 12 couldn't get here soon enough.

The day finally arrived, and the surgery couldn't have gone any better. I had no vomiting after the surgery, so I was able to go home after about an hour in the recovery room, although

I was quite nauseous. The surgery took longer than expected, but I was grateful that Dr. Sando took his time to make sure everything was exactly as it should be.

I needed some help removing my hospital gown and putting on a button-up shirt. Kurt helped, and as he took the gown off of me, he exclaimed, "Wow! They look amazing." We had joked that I would be getting "new boobs for Christmas." Apparently, he liked this Christmas present.

I experienced a great deal of pain for a few days after the surgery. I had incision scars across the center of each breast and all the way underneath my armpits almost to my back from removing the excess skin. I was so thankful to be rid of all of that skin, but the scars left behind were pretty significant. I was horrified to think that these scars would be with me for the rest of my days. I knew they would fade, but at the moment, they felt hideous to me. I wondered how anyone could find this body attractive. I kept these feelings hidden from Kurt, but I knew they would need to be addressed eventually.

Celebrating Christmas proved to be difficult. I was incredibly sore and had very limited range of motion in my arms. I wasn't able to attend any family Christmas gatherings because of the tenderness I still had in my chest, and I didn't want to take the chance of being bumped, jostled, or hugged.

Slowly but surely, physical healing came. Then it was time to deal with the emotional and psychological pain of cancer. Dealing with those issues would be another chapter in this seemingly never-ending journey. But I knew that with God, all things are possible. I knew He would remain faithful to me throughout.

PART II:

A BIBLICAL GUIDE TO
NAVIGATING LIFE AFTER CANCER

Chapter 1

CANCER-FREE — NOW WHAT?

What to Expect After Cancer

You've heard the diagnosis. You've been to all the doctors' appointments, had all the scans and labs, completed chemotherapy and radiation, and had surgery, if necessary. You've been through a whirlwind of activities where literally every second of every day of your life for months on end (or longer) was dictated by cancer. And suddenly, it's all over. Now what do you do? How do you navigate life after cancer?

Suddenly you have time on your hands. Maybe you're looking at going back to work. Maybe you're getting back into the groove of being a parent and a spouse. Maybe you are ready to start volunteering again. You're slightly excited and maybe a little reticent about starting out again. But you're struggling with a wave of emotions, and you're not sure what to do with all of them.

Most of the time, cancer patients are so busy simply trying to survive during treatment that they don't even have time to acknowledge or process the fact that they actually had feelings while going through treatment. Perhaps they had a wealth of support from family, friends, community, and their medical team. But once the treatments ended, they found themselves feeling incredibly alone and vulnerable. One of the hardest things to go through is not knowing what happens next.

When I completed the cancer treatment journey of eight cycles of chemotherapy in four months and then two surgeries, I felt like everything would be over and I would return to life as it was before. But I quickly realized that it wasn't over for me, and it's not over for many cancer patients. The side effects from chemo and surgeries can take weeks or longer to overcome, often leaving you feeling depleted for longer than you anticipated. To make matters worse, you may have lasting reminders of what you've been through such as scars or other physical issues, as well as emotional scars.

There are follow-up doctors' appointments. Many oncologists want to monitor you for a period of time before releasing you completely, if at all. You might have to have a scan or labs from time to time. That brings anxiety (also known as scanxiety) over a recurrence of cancer. Simply finding a lump or having a slight cough, a headache, or some other possible sign or symptom of cancer can cause anxiety and fear.

Now that you don't have the constant and almost daily interaction with your care team, you might wonder how to communicate with them or what questions to ask going forward. But now is not the time to shrink back in fear. If you haven't done so already, it's time to become your own health care advocate and work on keeping those lines of communication open with your doctor and care team. If you had a nurse navigator, as I did, use them. If you aren't scheduled for tests or an appointment with your oncologist and have a question, it's okay to check in with your nurse navigator. They're still your navigator even after your treatment is over.

I was afraid I would wear out my welcome with my nurse navigator. I had so many questions, but she always made herself available to me whenever I sent her an email, no matter how many months had passed since my last treatment. Together with your doctor, your nurse navigator will continue to make sure you have a good care plan in place for after-cancer care. And if no one suggests putting one in place, you should take the initiative and ask for one on your behalf. That will help you feel more secure in your after-cancer care and help you feel as if you are being involved in your own care as well. A wellness plan for after-cancer care should include your physical, emotional, social, and spiritual well-being. Don't be afraid to ask about all these categories of care.

Physical care might include how to cope with ongoing fatigue, nausea, pain, or even numbness or tingling in your extremities from chemotherapy. Part of helping you feel empowered might include making changes such as quitting smoking or drinking, starting to exercise or return to it, eating well, and having better sleep habits. Again, ask your medical team for tips on how to accomplish these goals.

Just as cancer can affect your physical health, it can also impact your emotional and spiritual health. Not only do you need to take care of your body after cancer treatments, but you also need to care well for your heart, mind, and soul. Not everyone will respond the same way to the trauma of surviving cancer. Different people from different walks of life will experience different emotions at different times. And that's okay. Don't compare yourself to others. Consider your own feelings first, and then consider a plan to address those issues. You might be dealing with some depression or anxiety. That could be addressed within the realm of your emotional care plan.

Talk with your pastor if you are struggling with anger at God or have questions about facing your own mortality due to a cancer diagnosis. That might include wondering how to ask for help from friends and family. Your doctor, a therapist, or a good pastor can help. Some cancer patients find themselves angry or bitter about what they've been through, while others experience intense grief over the things they've lost as a result of cancer. The gamut of emotions is wide and can feel just as overwhelming as the cancer journey itself. Feeling anger is normal. How you respond to that anger is what will make the biggest difference in your life. Hanging on to anger will hinder you from moving forward and healing entirely from your own cancer.

Perhaps you've found yourself the victim of cancer ghosting—someone you love disappears out of your life without reason after your cancer diagnosis. Perhaps you're left with questions about why they left you. Confusion abounds, and grief takes hold. Look at this as another opportunity to allow God to heal you from the inside out by addressing the issue with yourself. Consider what you want to happen with the relationship of the one who ghosted you, and then move forward with boundaries or goodbyes.

You may find yourself feeling lonely, especially if you had a strong support group while you were in the middle of your cancer journey. Reach out to the people who were there then. Let them know you miss them, and ask to grab a cup of coffee or lunch with them. Those people were there for you once before, and they'll be there again even as you recover emotionally. Consider joining a cancer support group in your community. Finding like-minded people who know what it's like to face cancer can help you feel less alone.

Maybe you're depressed. You survived. So why in the world are you depressed? Shouldn't you just be happy you survived? Yes. Well, sort of. You've been through a traumatic experience. It's important to acknowledge it. Let that thought sit with you for a while.

You've lost your hair, your strength, your stamina, and your sense of security. Your dreams, plans, and future may seem uncertain. You stared death in the face. It is perfectly normal to experience depression after facing such trauma. According to the American Cancer Society, one in four cancer patients will experience depression during or after treatment. You're not alone on this journey, and there are things you can do to find help and relief from depression.

- Talk about your feelings and fears with a trusted confidant or experienced counselor.
- Seek help through support groups or counseling.
- Ask about treatments for depression.
- Walking and breathing exercises can be helpful.
- Pray. Even if you don't know what to pray for, simply cry out to God. He hears, and He will answer. (Source: American Cancer Society)

Cancer is no respecter of age, race, hair color, creed, religion, or anything else. It strikes out of the blue and leaves us struggling. Eric Bobbitt, who is responsible for pastoral counseling and an elder with Zionsville Fellowship Church in Zionsville, Indiana, says that cancer is a great revealer of the human struggle and human questions. Here's what he said:

> Somehow, we convince ourselves that we can set certain questions aside or not deal with them now. Cancer strips that away. Why does God allow things to happen in the world? Why is this happening to me? What does this mean for me? What purpose does this have for my life? It brings grief and loss in huge ways along with fear, anxiety and anger. You come to the end of yourself, and you're pushed to a new dependency on God and on others in a way that you never have before.

The following chapters will tackle many of these questions and more. You'll find information on anger and bitterness, grief and depression, fear of recurrence of cancer, cancer ghosting, finding joy in the midst of suffering, intimacy in marriage after cancer surgery, why community and faith matter in the cancer journey, and even the gospel of Jesus Christ.

The end of treatment can be a time of fear, or you can allow it to bolster you into looking forward to the future. New beginnings can bring a sense of joy and relief. For me, cancer gave me a second chance to live life in a more meaningful and abundant way. I have an eternal perspective on my life as well as the lives of others around me. Coming to the conclusion of what works best for you will take time. Allow yourself that time to grieve, heal, and rejoice in a new beginning.

> *Beloved, Pray that all may go well with you and that you may be in good health, as it goes well with your soul.*
>
> —3 John 1:3

Deeper Still ...

1. Navigating life after cancer can be surprisingly difficult. Now that you've gone through and completed your cancer treatments, have you struggled with wondering what happens next? Explain what you're feeling or perhaps fearing.

2. It's vitally important to continue to be in communication with your care team, doctor, or nurse navigator in order to have a care plan in place for after-cancer care. Is this your experience? If not, you may consider reaching out and asking for one.

3. Cancer can leave you with not only physical scars but emotional scars. It's important to be honest and acknowledge these in order to move forward in your healing process. Take some time to be still and consider your heart, mind, and soul. Are you feeling anger, grief, loneliness, or depression? Consider talking openly and honestly with a counselor, support group, and especially your Creator God.

4. This chapter provided several suggestions concerning the battle of navigating life after cancer. From the following, what can you begin to apply today?

    a. Take time to ponder what truly matters, and rebuild your life around those things. Keep a journal, and write down what is giving you meaning in your life after cancer.

    b. Cling to the promises of truth, hope, and eternity. Pray that God will give you an eternal perspective.

    c. Allow yourself time to grieve, heal, and rejoice in a new beginning.

Chapter 2

EMOTIONS AND CANCER: ANGER AND BITTERNESS

Never doubt a mother's intuition. Jackson had the flu. But when symptoms persisted and new ones arose, Kristina was quick to take action for her 18-year-old son. He had a cough that lasted longer than it should have. He was feverish and lost vocal strength and stamina when he sang with his high school show choir. And then he started passing out. In three weeks, Jackson had lost about 40 pounds.

Kristina took him to his pediatrician where "give it time" was the prescription. Emergency room visits became regular occurrences for the Williams family, often taking place in the evening when Jackson suffered the most. Jackson's father, Greg, told his son that one more bad night would mean another trip to the ER. Jackson resisted because no one could figure out what was wrong with him, and he didn't think anyone would ever be able to find the answer. But Kristina and Greg insisted. And when

Jackson was taken to the hospital at 4:30 one morning, Kristina insisted that the staff take a chest X-ray. This was after weeks of unanswered questions from ER doctors and Jackson's pediatrician.

The X-ray showed a large mass the size of a football growing in Jackson's chest. Because of the way it was positioned near the heart, one of his main arteries was being impacted and squeezed, which caused him to pass out regularly. The emergency room doctor initially said it was Hodgkin lymphoma. More invasive testing showed that Jackson had non-Hodgkin lymphoma called T-cell lymphoblastic lymphoma (TLL).

The Williams family was initially grateful and relieved with an answer to their many questions. And Jackson was grateful for his mother's advocacy on his behalf. "I wasn't able to function properly, so how am I supposed to advocate for myself?" he said of his mother's help.

Once reality set in, there was a whole new set of emotions. Kristina was grateful for the speed in how the medical community began Jackson's care, but she wondered if he would survive. Jackson dreaded the thought of the two and a half years of treatment he would face.

Jackson was in his senior year of high school, and he was finishing strong in academics and the show choir. He would miss out on so much, including graduation. It would also mean missing out on his first year at Purdue University where he planned to study mechanical engineering.

"My life was about to change for a long time," Jackson said, "and so there were a lot of emotions. I think there was some relief just to have a diagnosis, but I was probably at the lowest of lows I had been."

He was immediately sent to Riley Children's Hospital in Indianapolis, Indiana. He went through multiple bone marrow biopsies and was immediately started on chemotherapy and steroids. He remained at Riley for 60 days getting various chemo treatments. The good news was that his type of mass was fast-growing, which also meant it would be fast-shrinking. But he knew there would be a long road ahead of him.

In the hospital, Jackson had plenty of time to think, especially since he was mostly isolated from friends and his sister, Eva, who wasn't yet old enough to visit him in the hospital. "I definitely missed having the opportunity to finish out my last year in school," Jackson said. "Senior year is closing out a chapter of your life, so I was pretty disappointed to be in the hospital. I was also starting to think about how my friends were going to be at college while I had to be at home. I tried to implement my faith for how I was framing the situation, but it wasn't always easy."

A severe drug shortage hit the hospital where Jackson was being treated, and it directly impacted his treatment. The only place Jackson could continue his treatment was at Children's Hospital of Philadelphia. He was there for five months, staying in an apartment with his father, away from family and friends. It was there that he found himself more isolated. He became bitter and angry. He explained, "Philly for sure was a dark time just because a lot of things weren't working out for me. I think when you start to lose your grip on your mental space or physical space, it makes it really hard spiritually to maintain optimism. It was just a void for me where I couldn't see a lot of light for a long time. I think the isolation didn't help at all, either."

Jackson found that he didn't want to be associated or connected with his feelings any longer. He distanced himself from the Lord during that dark time. He wanted to get to the end of his treatments and forget it all happened.

Once Jackson returned home and began maintenance medicine, he found a connection with some friends who had been together in a small group at church for many years. The group of young men was younger than Jackson, but he was compelled to join. "It was really important for me to start to refocus on my faith and just rekindle that fire for the Lord because it was lost for a while," he said. He also went through some counseling to help him connect with the strong emotions that had kept him in a dark place for such a long period of time.

Jackson says he was finally able to move on once he was able to enter his first year of college. "I closed off a lot of feelings and emotions that maybe I wasn't always used to expressing," he said. "I think I got bitter from my experience even though I was happy to have some normalcy. There was definitely a part of me that had changed dramatically." He said counseling helped with that and allowed him to dig deep to open his heart again. Reprioritizing his faith was also a key to healing from the losses he experienced.

Feelings of anger are common among cancer patients. Those feelings can crop up anytime during or after treatments. And those feelings are completely normal. It is a normal response for patients after first being diagnosed, but it is also common for those who suffer a recurrence of cancer.

Anger often comes from feelings that are hard to show. For example, anger can stem from feelings of sadness, fear, frustration, anxiety, or helplessness. The anger cancer patients experience is no different than the anger in any other crisis, such as the loss of a loved one. Some people see anger as a negative emotion, but it can often be quite positive.

"Some patients can take the anger and say, 'I'm going to use this to fight back,'" said Dr. Philip Bialer, a psychiatrist at Memorial Sloan Kettering Cancer Center in New York.[1] But for cancer patients to use it to their advantage, they must recognize the anger and acknowledge it. One way to do so is through counseling or group therapy. Therapy has shown to improve quality of life and can help reduce anxiety and depression, which are also common emotions when faced with cancer.

Not everyone will experience anger during cancer treatments. Some people don't experience anger until after the treatments are over. Such was the case for Debbie Woodbury who received a breast cancer diagnosis in 2009. She had a mastectomy, and her treatment was successful. However, she shared that she had a hard time getting back to life as usual. She discovered that she was angry. "I was dealing with what I had gone through, what I had lost, and what I now knew about my mortality," Debbie said. "And that brought up a lot of resentment and anger."[2]

There are myriad reasons to feel angry, including the following:

- The difficult journey you have just experienced through treatments or surgeries.
- Unsupportive friends or family members, including those who ghost you (see Chapter 5).

- The side-effects of treatments.
- A negative experience with a doctor or nurse.
- Changes to your life because of cancer, such as a pause to parenting or a career.
- Not being able to do as much as before due to fatigue or pain.
- Other people being in good health.
- Events you may have missed out on due to your treatment or surgery recovery time.
- The impact cancer has had on relationships.

Many people, believer and nonbeliever alike, often find themselves angry with God. This is also completely normal. It's important to face anger and bitterness head on before it festers within you and creates other issues. Ask yourself, *Where do my anger and bitterness fit in?* And then consider how to address it. Perhaps most importantly, address it with God.

"If you're bitter, be bitter," said Bob Ash who is responsible for pastoral care at Zionsville Fellowship Church in Zionsville, Indiana. "Be honest. Don't try to beat yourself up for being bitter and angry. But don't beat up other people over your anger either." Letting God know how you feel is a key component in dealing with those emotions.

"If you're a Christian, God already knows you're upset," said Ash. "Why not just tell Him? And then examine why you're bitter or angry. Ask yourself if it [the anger] is valid."

Ash recommends searching your heart to see who or what is making you angry. Are you angry at God? The medical establishment? People in your life who aren't sick?

"If it's valid, be bitter and angry. Just don't stay there for the rest of your life," Ash said.

In addition to examining your own heart, Ash recommends digging into who God says He is. "Ask yourself what you believe about God," he said. "What believing in God does is give you hope to deal with the things that have entered your life. If you think of what faith can give you in hope and encouragement, those are the things that will replace your bitterness and anger over time. But it's not going to happen overnight."

So then, how do you cope with anger? Many people will take advantage of counseling. Another tool for dealing with anger is journaling. Writing your feelings down can be incredibly cathartic. Connecting with emotions through the art of writing can be very helpful. Even if you're not skilled as a writer, write it down anyway. Allow yourself to pour out your emotions on paper or on a computer. Focus on the things you've lost or how you felt during or after treatment. Write down whatever comes to your mind. Don't stifle whatever pops into your thoughts. You may feel anger rise up in you as you write, but continue the writing process. Getting in touch with those emotions is a great way to release the anger from inside of you. You'll probably notice a sensation of feeling free when you have completed your writing. Sit with that feeling of freedom for a while and let it wash over you.

If you're not sure about writing down what you're feeling, start a gratitude journal. There is no way you can be angry when you're thankful. You may ask, "What do I have to be thankful for?" If you're uncertain, try the ABC method of gratitude. Go through the alphabet and write down one thing you're grateful for with each letter. For the letter A, you might be grateful for the "Ability to spend time with friends or family." For the letter B, you might write that you can "Bring joy to others by sending an encouraging text message even when you're not feeling the best." And so on. You can even use the ABC method when thanking God for certain people who were there for you during your darkest days. I wrote down that I was thankful for Amy, Becky, Cinda, Deb, and more. You can go through the entire alphabet.

Another way to cope with anger is to use your voice. Vocalize your emotions with someone who will listen unconditionally and without condemnation. Don't direct your anger at a person but use the physical action of transferring sound as a method of letting go. What does that look like outside of talking to a friend? Try screaming into a pillow or yelling in a private and safe space such as in your car. You can also try singing as loudly as you can to a high-intensity song. Singing praise and worship music is bound to change your mood because the focus is on the Lord instead of your circumstances.

Consider praying and meditating on Scripture. If you're not even sure how to utter a prayer, try the ABC method for praying. Praise God for who He is with words of His character. A for Almighty, B for Bright morning star, C for Comforter, and so on. Pray the Psalms to remember God's goodness and mercy. Meditate on the promises of God. Use a Bible app or Biblegateway.com for help with topical scriptures.

Moving your body is another way to cope with anger. Exercising during and after cancer is beneficial to the healing of your body. It not only releases anger but calms your mind. Take a brisk walk. Consider running if you're strong enough. Cycle. Swim if you have access to a swimming pool. Dancing or circuit training can be another fun way to release anger. Exercise wasn't an option for me during my treatments because I was so weak and had no stamina. But once chemo was over, I began working out with a personal trainer who has helped me regain my strength. Putting my physical and mental energy into pulling or lifting weights allowed me to release negative thoughts that had been bottled up inside of me for months due to treatment and surgeries.

Despite working out for many months with a personal trainer, a trip to England with my husband showed me that I still had a long way to go in my recovery. I wasn't able to keep up with my husband and had to pause on long walks or bike rides. I became angry that cancer had stolen my stamina. But I had to remind myself that getting cancer wasn't my fault. I had to give myself grace on the journey and not beat myself up for where I was in my recovery. Recognizing that my body had been through a major trauma and was still in recovery allowed me to bend a little in my anger. A good cry here and there also showed me the benefits of releasing the emotions I had stuffed deep inside during my treatments.

In those moments of frustration, I asked myself what I was really angry about. Giving myself an honest answer helped free me from the initial outburst of anger. But I also had to reframe the way I talked to myself. Instead of saying, "I can't do this anymore," I reminded myself that I may be weak now and perhaps can't do as much as I used to, but it's a temporary situation. I am doing things every day to strengthen my body and am working as hard as my body will allow to change my circumstances. Reframing the way you talk to yourself is a great coping tool.

Another trigger for anger is the fear of recurrence. I suspect nearly every cancer survivor fears the recurrence of their cancer. One way to help combat that fear and subsequent anger is to schedule regular visits with your cancer care team. Get your blood work checked regularly. Have scans if your insurance allows for it. Talk with your medical team about your fears and how to handle them. If your fears are overwhelming and you can't seem to shake them, you may want to consider counseling to learn how to reframe your thinking about the recurrence of cancer. Here are some other ways to combat the fear of recurrence.

- *Be informed:* Learn as much as you can about your type of cancer. Learn about services where you can find support and stay informed.
- *Have a positive attitude:* Don't automatically allow yourself to think the worst in every situation. Focus on wellness and the things that are going right in your life right now.
- *Find ways to relax:* Take a hot bath. Enjoy a brisk walk in the park. Snuggle with a pet. Listen to soothing music. Read a good book.
- *Be active:* Don't allow yourself to be stuck inside as you ruminate over what could be wrong. Get out and enjoy time with friends and family.

- *Control what you can:* You can't control when your body gets cancer, but you can control making regular doctors' appointments, focusing on your own wellness, and making lifestyle changes where necessary.

Feel what you're feeling in its entirety. But always take the necessary steps to overcome the anger and bitterness. Eric Bobbitt explained it this way:

> I think one of the first and most important things is you have to feel what you feel. But when you come face to face with all the losses of cancer, you have to deal with them, or you will be bitter, angry, grouchy, miserable. And so will everyone around you. You've got to step right into the storm, all the losses, and face the reality of those things with the wisdom of the ages with the Scripture and with people that love you and even go through it with people who have gone through it before you.

Finally, don't sin in your anger. Don't take it out on other people, especially those closest to you. If you find yourself snapping or yelling at someone you love, offer an apology and find more constructive ways to communicate your anger. Also, remember the promises of God (see Appendix B, The Promises of God). Remember who God is. If you're unsure of the character of God, see Appendix A (The Character of God) to learn who God is. If you're a survivor, remember that the Lord brought you to healing once already. Give thanks and focus on that instead of what angers you about having had cancer in the first place. Trust that God does have your best interest at heart and will only allow those things in your life that will serve to change you into the likeness of His Son and glorify Him. Trust in the goodness of our great God.

Deeper Still ...

1. After reading this chapter of another's journey with cancer, what feelings or emotions are you experiencing as you recall your own journey?

2. Experiencing anger during or even after cancer is very common. If that has been (or is now) your experience, write down your thoughts and feelings.

3. Bitterness and anger are not negative emotions. Even the Lord Jesus experienced anger, sadness, fear, and frustration. Spend some time being still, and ask yourself if there is someone or something that has caused you to be bitter or angry on your cancer journey. Record your thoughts.

4. After identifying who or what you may be angry about, read the definitions below. If you have sinned in your anger, ask the Lord for His forgiveness.

   Sin: Lawlessness (1 John 3:4) or transgression of God's will, either by not doing what God's law requires or doing what it forbids. The transgression can occur in thought (1 John 3:15), word (Matt. 5:22), or deed (Rom. 1:32).

   Forgiveness: The act of excusing or pardoning another in spite of their slights, shortcomings, and errors. As a theological term, forgiveness refers to God's pardon of the sins of human beings (1 John 1:9).

5. During or after your journey with cancer, did you find yourself angry with God, questioning His goodness and love for you? If so, He understands and welcomes you with open arms to come to Him and share your feelings. Take time to sit in silence and be honest with yourself and with God.

6. After completing this chapter and the Deeper Still questions, what have you learned about your journey with cancer, yourself, and God?

Chapter 3

EMOTIONS AND CANCER: GRIEF AND DEPRESSION

It felt like it happened in a split second. I was fine one second, and the next I felt a tsunami of emotion sweep over me. I had no idea what was happening to me or how to stop it. All I knew was that I couldn't stop it, and I had no control over my feelings.

Although chemotherapy was in the rearview mirror by nearly a year and both surgeries were completed, I was still taking naps every afternoon. My body was riddled with fatigue and a lack of energy from chemotherapy, and what I didn't know at the time was that I had an iron deficiency due to chemotherapy. Naps were a lifeline to get me through the days of continued healing. Once when I felt the wave come over me, I was scrolling online senselessly after a nap. My mother, who was now living with us, was downstairs getting her afternoon cappuccino. I couldn't put a finger on what was happening to me. I just knew I needed to cry. I put my phone on the bed, rolled over, and buried my face in a pillow. The tears flowed freely, and I almost threw up from the intensity of the emotion. Suddenly the tears stopped as quickly as they had started. But I felt a heaviness in my heart that I hadn't felt in years.

I was no stranger to depression. I'd had an intimate relationship with it since my early 20s. And then I was diagnosed with post-traumatic stress disorder after my close encounter with 9/11. Thankfully, the Lord chose to heal me of PTSD-related depression. I hadn't had a depressive episode since 2015—that is, until that moment when the tears flowed.

But why? Sure, I'd had cancer. But I was cancer-free now. I was putting the chemo and surgery behind me. I was still trying to get back to normal. The Lord kept putting a word on my heart: *grief*. I was confused, so I just continued to pray. Why? What was I grieving? How could I be grieving when I'd had a successful outcome from a cancer diagnosis? As I prayed, the Lord confirmed some things I hadn't thought about.

From the moment of my diagnosis, I was on the fast train to treatment. All I knew was that I had to buckle up and get ready for the ride of a lifetime. And it wasn't going to be a fun ride either. I was shuffled from scans to doctors' appointments, to chemo, to the couch, to bed, to blood draws, to day-after shots, to everything cancer-related. It was a whirlwind, and I didn't know what was coming next. My friend Tana, whose own daughter Haley had faced a long battle with leukemia, used to tell me, "Do the next thing." I later learned that this was from a poem popularized by the late missionary and author Elisabeth

Elliot. And that was literally all I could do during my cancer journey—the next thing.

But that next thing didn't involve or include dealing with the myriad emotions of what was happening to me. Never once during my treatment did I have time to sit and reflect on what I was feeling or how I felt about a breast cancer diagnosis. Cancer didn't allow for such luxuries as time to reflect. Now that cancer was silent, I had time—lots of time. Suddenly and without warning, the first emotion I had to deal with came in the form of grief.

No one told me this would happen. No one told me to expect grief to come in such a catastrophic manner. I never knew that various emotions might eventually join in on the assault of my mind and heart. But here was grief. And I was alone with it for days before I finally figured out what it was. And by then, the grief was almost overwhelming.

I didn't tell anyone, not even my husband. I felt like such a burden with this added issue. I felt like I needed to explore what was happening inside me before I revealed it to anyone. It started out by recognizing that I had cancer fatigue. Everywhere I looked (Facebook, Instagram, TV, books), something about breast cancer or cancer in general was thrown in my face. Advertisements for mastectomy bras or how to know if you have breast cancer were everywhere. There were support groups, research groups, genetic testing, and all types of breast cancer ads. It was a constant barrage of images and information, and it was overwhelming. I began to feel as if I were in the midst of the battle again before realizing that this was a continuation of the battle. Cancer is not only a disease of the body but also a battle of the mind.

I continued with the grief deep within me without telling a soul for many months. By the time I did share it with others, I was knee-deep into writing my own book about navigating life after cancer. I had a group of women who had committed to pray for me through the writing process, and I felt it was necessary to share my feelings with them in order to begin the healing process. I also realized that this was part of a story that needed to be told for the benefit of others. Of course, those women, ever faithful, did pray for me. My nurse navigator connected me with a counselor who has more than a decade of experience in palliative care with cancer patients. She has been absolutely amazing in helping me process grief and so many other emotions I wasn't expecting to have. I also shared this with my husband who, also ever faithful, promised to pray for me and walk through this part of the journey with me as well.

So then, what exactly is grief? Tim Challies, author of many books, including one about his journey through the painful loss of his son and how God comforted him through that journey, wrote in *Seasons of Sorrow*, " Is grief an emotion or a feeling? Is it a thing or a being? Could it be a state or sin, an origin or a destination? I am coming to understand grief as a response and a process—a response to circumstances and a process that begins with a sore trial or deep loss. And while I am less certain of the destination, I think it must be acceptance, submission, peace and hope."[3]

Bob Ash says, "I think that in grief, if you look at grief as a process, not an event, grief takes time. Grief can take a lifetime. You don't forget stuff. I don't forget the saddest parts of things that have happened to me, but I don't dwell on them."

My dear friend and mentor suggested that I name the things I was grieving. Calling them by name would allow me to become intimately familiar with them and know how to process the feelings attached to them. So I began the process of writing down what I was grieving. I didn't realize there were so many things I was grieving over.

For example, I felt I had lost my innocence to cancer. It wasn't that I had been shielded from cancer—my father had died from small cell carcinoma—but I was shielded from it happening to *me*. And now cancer was part of my story, my history, and my every single day whether it was in the form of the book I was writing, thoughts and fears of recurrence, or just remembering what I had gone through.

Before my cancer diagnosis, I was heavily involved in various ministries at church. After my diagnosis, I had to leave the writing team, and I wasn't able to spend time preparing for lectures. Our Bible study was over by the time I was in the middle of cancer treatments. I missed quite a few Missions Team meetings. I missed out on so much because of cancer, and I'll never get those moments of ministry back. I wondered why was so much of my ministry was seemingly being taken away from me.

In the middle of my cancer journey, I was blessed by many wonderful people—some I didn't know well—who came to visit me and keep me company in the off weeks of my chemotherapy treatments. Once chemo was over, I found myself alone—no more visitors. People didn't disappear or stop caring. I just missed the companionship that had been almost a daily part of my life. And that was another reason to grieve.

I was also grieving the great disappointment I had in family members who completely ignored my cancer diagnosis. I fully expected some of them to be there, and they were and are still nowhere to be found. I later learned that this is called cancer ghosting (see Chapter 5). At the moment, those relationships seem beyond salvageable, but I know that with God, all things are possible. Only He knows what could come of these seemingly tattered relationships. In the meantime, there is a sense of loss followed by grief for what could have and should have been.

In the process of going through chemotherapy, I lost everything that made me feminine, including my breasts. I was deeply grieving those losses as well.

Those are just some of the ways I felt loss and ultimately went through a period of deep grieving. My friend suggested that we undertake an exercise of processing these losses from a spiritual perspective. Her idea was to focus on what Scripture says about what we as believers can and must do when faced with difficulties in life. She reminded me of some verses in Ephesians and Colossians where the Apostle Paul admonishes believers to put off their old self and put on the new self. Let's take a look at these verses that are so critical in the rethinking of loss and grief.

> *Now this I say and testify in the Lord, that you must no longer walk as the Gentiles do, in the futility of their minds. They are darkened in their understanding, alienated from the life of God because of the ignorance that is in them, due to*

their hardness of heart. They have become callous and have given themselves up to sensuality, greedy to practice every kind of impurity. But that is not the way you learned Christ!—assuming that you have heard about him and were taught in him, as the truth is in Jesus, to put off your old self, which belongs to your former manner of life and is corrupt through deceitful desires, and to be renewed in the spirit of your minds, and to put on the new self, created after the likeness of God in true righteousness and holiness. Therefore, having put away falsehood, let each one of you speak the truth with his neighbor, for we are members one of another. Be angry and do not sin; do not let the sun go down on your anger, and give no opportunity to the devil. Let the thief no longer steal, but rather let him labor, doing honest work with his own hands, so that he may have something to share with anyone in need. Let no corrupting talk come out of your mouths, but only such as is good for building up, as fits the occasion, that it may give grace to those who hear. And do not grieve the Holy Spirit of God, by whom you were sealed for the day of redemption. Let all bitterness and wrath and anger and clamor and slander be put away from you, along with all malice. Be kind to one another, tenderhearted, forgiving one another, as God in Christ forgave you.

—Eph. 4:17–32

Put on then, as God's chosen ones, holy and beloved, compassionate hearts, kindness, humility, meekness, and patience, bearing with one another and, if one has a complaint against another, forgiving each other; as the Lord has forgiven you, so you also must forgive. And above all these put on love, which binds everything together in perfect harmony. And let the peace of Christ rule in your hearts, to which indeed you were called in one body. And be thankful. Let the word of Christ dwell in you richly, teaching and admonishing one another in all wisdom, singing psalms and hymns and spiritual songs, with thankfulness in your hearts to God. And whatever you do, in word or deed, do everything in the name of the Lord Jesus, giving thanks to God the Father through him.

—Col. 3:12–17

Ray Stedman, in his daily devotional (raystedman.org), explains these verses in greater detail:

Putting off the old and putting on the new is the principle by which the possibilities that are in Christ can become evident in our experience. Notice there is a recognition of the pull of the old life on the Christian. The admonition of the apostle is to be constantly recognizing and rejecting these false, underlying assumptions that come from the old self, the old way of living. It is not merely deeds, you will notice, but outlooks and attitudes. This is what causes the problem, and this is what we must reject.

Put off means to divest yourself of something, to take it off. Paul is using the simplest of terms to illustrate what we must do in the realm of thought, of the attitudes of life. We must reject those basic assumptions that have caused our trouble—putting them off, rejecting them, divesting ourselves of them—just as you would put off your dirty clothes.

We must do this because the corruption of life comes from these wrong attitudes. Paul says the former manner of life is corrupt—decayed, dead, foul, selfish, unhappy, restless. These are the things that have made life unhappy or miserable. He points out we can recognize these attitudes by the way they operate. They are deceitful lusts. Unfortunately, this word lust is greatly misunderstood in our day. We invariably associate it with something sexual. But this word is much broader than that. It means any urge or basic drive. We will get closer to the essential meaning of this word if we use the term urge. These deceitful urges are constantly coming to us as we react to various situations in which we find ourselves.

The first step in experiencing what God intends for us is to recognize that. Put off the old. That is the first step. The other is to recognize the wonderful possibilities of the new life. In that phrase, to be made new in the attitude of your minds, you have the fundamental difference between a Christian and a non-Christian. It is true that non-Christians sometimes realize that things are wrong in their lives, and so they change them. But they merely change to another expression of the same basic egocentricity. They change the outer form, but the problem remains basically the same.

But of all human beings, Christians alone have the possibility of doing something entirely different, living by an entirely different principle, because they have been renewed in the attitude of their minds. And that happens in the regenerated life as the Spirit of God comes into the heart that believes in Jesus Christ. When we believe in Jesus Christ and receive Him as our Lord and Savior, we are renewed in the attitudes of our minds. The new self is in the likeness of God: it is the life of God; it is the image of Jesus Christ; it is His life lived in you. So put on that kind of life, because it is available to you.

What does this look like where grief is concerned? My friend took me through each of the losses and griefs I shared, and asked what I was holding onto in each of the losses. For example, take the loss of innocence I felt. Here is what I discovered about my beliefs and what I needed to "put off" before I could "put on" new thoughts about that loss.

Put off old thoughts: I had to put to death the idea that I was impervious to cancer. As I have discovered, everyone is susceptible to cancer. And it can strike at any time and without warning. I keep trying to return to the old ways of life, as if returning to normal will somehow make it all go away as if it never happened. But I've also discovered that normal isn't normal anymore. And going back isn't possible.

Put on new thoughts: Cancer is part of my everyday life now. I'm getting used to it, and the innocence I lost is forever gone. I'm accepting that slowly but surely. I simply need to remember the faithfulness of God. He was with me in the midst of cancer, He will be with me (and is with me) in the aftermath of cancer. He was faithful to me then, He will continue to be faithful to me now, even if the cancer returns. But I simply can't live in the *what ifs*. I need to rest in the promises He has made to me and enjoy the gift of another chance at life, no matter how long it may last, and make the most of what time I have on this earth.

Going through this process for each of the losses I shared helped me see how to process and navigate through those emotions to the point where the intensity of the grief began to wane and I wasn't stuck in a cycle of pain and searing loss. It was a remarkable experience of healing, and I recommend it to you if you are struggling with loss and grief.

Before we explore other ways to cope with grief, let's dig deeper into the symptoms of grief. According to the University of Rochester Medical Center, grief can include physical symptoms, emotional symptoms, and spiritual symptoms. That doesn't mean you'll experience all of them at one time.

Physical symptoms can include fatigue, lack of energy, headaches, upset stomach, excessive sleeping, overworking, or being involved in too many activities. Emotional symptoms can include memory lapses, distraction, preoccupation, irritability, depression, feelings of euphoria, extreme anger, or feelings of being resigned to the situation. Spiritual symptoms can include feelings of being closer to God, anger and outrage at God, strengthening your faith, or questioning your faith.

The grieving process is different for everyone, and not everyone follows the same path of grieving. It also doesn't last the same amount of time for everyone. The stages of grief don't happen in any particular order, and sometimes not all the stages are included in the process. The five stages of grief include denial, anger, bargaining, depression and sadness, and acceptance.

Alan D. Wolfelt, PhD, wrote an article called "The Grief and Mourning of Cancer" for *Coping with Cancer* magazine. He says grief is natural after you have learned what it means to be healthy one moment and are suddenly unhealthy the next. "Grief is what we think and feel on the inside when we lose someone or something important," wrote Wolfelt. "We experience shock, anger, guilt, sadness and other emotions." And he says grief requires mourning. "While grief is what's bottled up inside you, mourning is the opening up, the letting out, and the sharing. … Without mourning, grief festers. If it is not expressed fully and honestly, it tends to result in ongoing problems."[5]

The American Cancer Society website says there are different ways to cope with grief. The list below is based on that advice, shortened and paraphrased a bit for ease of reading.

- Let your feelings out. Let yourself experience your feelings. Don't judge yourself for those feelings. They are completely normal.
- Be patient. Let your grief happen at its own pace. Don't judge yourself against how someone else is grieving.

- Find ways to be creative. Seek out a music or art therapist, or write your thoughts and feelings in a journal.
- Take care of yourself. Try to get enough sleep, eat a healthy diet, and exercise regularly.
- Keep up your routine. Having a daily routine helps you know what to do with yourself and your time.
- Talk with other loved ones. Let them help you through the process.
- Enjoy time with family and friends. It's okay to give yourself a break from the grieving process. Give yourself permission to go and enjoy yourself.[6]

Finally, spend time with God. Open the Bible and read the Psalms to encourage your heart. There you'll find others who have been through the grieving process, and you'll see how they carried on by faith. There are other passages in Scripture that talk about grief and how to cope. (See Appendix C, Scriptures for Dealing with Grief.) Take time to pray. Even if all you can mutter is "help me," then say it. And say it again. Sing songs of worship and gratitude. It's not about trying to dismiss what you're facing. It's about trying to shift your focus to God's incredible and tender mercies that are new every day.

Deeper Still ...

1. Have you experienced the physical, emotional, or spiritual symptoms of grief? If so, explain your experience using as many words as you can to describe what you thought or felt.

2. It can be challenging, even scary, to allow yourself to feel and fully experience the emotions God has given us. If you find this to be true as you think about grief and depression, be patient with yourself. God understands and will walk with you through the process of acceptance, submission, peace, and hope. If He has been faithful to do this for you in the past, how might remembering those times help during your process now?

3. Sharing with a trusted friend or family member all that you may be feeling can create a healthy honesty in your relationship. Who is that person you can be open with regarding your deepest feelings? Pray that God will open doors for conversations with that person.

4. From the Scriptures provided in this chapter, which ones did you find most helpful?

5. Are there other passages in the Bible that were an encouragement to you during or after your time of grief and depression?

6. How could this chapter be helpful in coming alongside someone else who may be experiencing grief or depression?

Chapter 4

EMOTIONS AND CANCER: FEAR OF RECURRENCE

One of the happiest and most joyful days of your cancer journey will be when you get to ring the bell after chemotherapy or radiation treatments come to an end. Ringing the bell means for some that they are cancer-free. But generally, it means that your cancer treatments have finally come to an end. For me, it was a celebration that rivaled every celebration I'd ever had.

If you remember my story in the Introduction to Part I, you'll recall my overwhelming joy when I got to ring that bell, when my husband and my mother celebrated with me, when the nursing staff cheered, and when my family and friends in the parking lot hooted and hollered as I walked outside. The announcement that I was cancer-free would come soon, and my bilateral mastectomy would finally be over. I was filled with joy and elation for several weeks despite the pain and fatigue. But then something inside of me changed.

I remember exactly where I was when the fear of recurrence of cancer hit me. I was visiting with my oncologist for my first three-month checkup following treatment. Labs showed that my calcium numbers were elevated, which caused my oncologist some concern. More tests couldn't pinpoint the reason for the high numbers. She recommended a scan to see if the cancer had returned, this time to my bones. She never said that's what she was looking for, but I knew that's what she was looking for. She had warned that if the cancer returned, it would be in the bones, the brain, the liver, or the lungs. And here I was thinking about a recurrence of cancer possibly in the bones just months after I was told there was no evidence of the disease. I was terrified. Thankfully, the scan showed no signs of cancer, but the fear didn't end with that bit of good news.

I quickly learned that fear of recurrence is very common among cancer patients who are in remission. In fact, the American Cancer Society estimates that at least 70 percent of survivors experience this type of fear. It can be powerful and negatively impact your quality of life if it is left unchecked. But why do we survivors even go there?

There are multiple factors that can influence fear of recurrence. Your specific history and diagnosis may cause this fear to rise up in you. It may happen, for example, if you have had a family history of cancer and then are diagnosed with it yourself. Sometimes cancer patients are given statistics (as I was) predicting the potential of recurrence, or there has been genetic testing to see if there is a gene mutation lurking, as I have. Perhaps you had a cancer particularly hard to treat or one that is very aggressive. Other triggers include certain events, anniversaries, or activities that could remind you of your cancer and cause you to start wondering if it will return. Even a new diagnosis for a friend or acquaintance might trigger your fear of recurrence.

The anniversary of your diagnosis or the beginning or end of treatment could be a day of celebration, or it could bring back difficult memories. The emotions and fears you felt those first days could come flooding back into your mind, sparking more fears of the cancer returning.

Non-occasions such as words, sights, tastes, sounds, or smells might spark fear in you. You may smell something that reminds you of the infusion room where you received your treatment. Perhaps you see a woman wearing a headscarf and remember when you had to don one yourself. You may be flooded in your social media feed with news, images, or articles about cancer that remind you of your own journey. That could bring back negative emotions and cause fear to rise up in you.

Physical symptoms can also cause a fear of recurrence. Symptoms such as fatigue or a headache, pain, cough, or other sensation that you associate with cancer might generate fear. Where physical symptoms come into play, some oncologists operate on a two-week rule. If any pain or symptom persists after two weeks, it should be checked. However, that doesn't mean you should wait two full weeks before contacting your medical team, especially if something is quite alarming.

You may find that you worry more about your cancer returning when it's time for a follow-up health care appointment, scans, blood tests, or other medical procedures. You might be concerned when you hear or read something about cancer that frightens you. Your most intense fears may come while you are waiting for test results. Scanxiety is a real thing for cancer survivors. Depending on your personality, you may tend to prepare for the worst while hoping for the best. To ensure your results come quickly, you may want to avoid scheduling tests right before a weekend or a holiday.

Sometimes the end of treatment may cause an uncertain fear because you have lost a regular connection with your medical care team. Instead of seeing them daily or weekly, you are now required to check in only once every few months. That may cause you to feel a sense of loss of control over your health and perhaps a belief that your medical team isn't staying on top of your care as much as when you were in the middle of treatment.

This was the case for Sarah. At the young age of 37, she was diagnosed with invasive lobular breast cancer, stage 2B. She had no history of breast cancer in her family, so it came as a complete shock. She went through chemotherapy, radiation, and a bilateral mastectomy. When the day came for her to ring the bell, she discovered that she wasn't as excited as she thought she should be.

"It was really scary to stop [treatment]," she reflected. "What if there's still something in there, and maybe I need a little more?" Sarah says that for her, fear of recurrence isn't all-consuming, but she admits that there isn't a day that goes by that she doesn't think about cancer in some form. And when she allows herself to think about the statistics, which are frightening, she reminds herself that there is also a high percentage that the cancer won't come back.

According to LiveStrong, fear of recurrence may become problematic for the cancer survivor for a variety of reasons.

- Any minor aches, coughs, or headaches that bring on a strong fear cancer has recurred.
- There is an unwillingness to rebuild and return to a full life due to fears.
- Recurrence is a constant worry.
- You have thoughts of the cancer returning right before you go to bed or first thing in the morning or both.
- Long-term sleep problems (lasting longer than a few weeks).
- Little or no appetite for days.
- No desire to spend time with family or friends.
- No interest in usual routines.

People respond to these fears in different ways. Some seek out reassurance and require extra visits with their oncologist. Some request additional screenings or other tests, engage in overtreatment, or excessively examine their bodies for signs of recurrence. On the other end of the spectrum, people resort to avoidance, including skipping or delaying follow-up visits, engaging in substance abuse, or hiding out in sedentary behavior or social isolation.

Living with uncertainty is never easy. Most cancer survivors worry most about the recurrence of cancer during the first year after treatment. That worry begins to wane after the first year. There are ways to cope with fears of recurrence.

First, don't ignore your fears. Accept that you are going to have these fears, and focus on ways to manage anxiety. My therapist, Melissa, even suggests allowing yourself to stay with your thoughts of fear for a short period of time. She says to give yourself a set amount of time to allow your mind to consider the possibilities of the recurrence of cancer. Let the thoughts fill your mind and contemplate how you would respond if the cancer did return. Once the timer goes off, move on to other thoughts, including things that remind you of the truth of your situation.

"I have to focus on the facts," explains Sarah. "My brain wants to go to the scary places. But I have to say to myself, 'You don't have stage 4 cancer; you had stage 2 cancer. And it's out now. It's gone. I'm healthy. My body is strong.' I have to focus on the here and now, and the other thoughts are simply not true."

There are other ways to combat the fear of recurrence. Let's start with talking.

"Don't keep it in," says Sarah. "I have to talk about it. Taking it to God, praying about it, giving the Lord my fears, talking to my family, talking to my friends. Because if you try to keep it in, it just grows, and it gives it more power."

Talking to the Lord is of the utmost importance. As Sarah says, we have to give our fears over to the Lord. The Psalms and 1 Peter remind us that we can take our fears to Him who hears and answers.

I sought the LORD, and he answered me and delivered me from all my fears.

—Ps. 34:4

Humble yourselves, therefore, under the mighty hand of
God so that at the proper time he may exalt you, casting
all your anxiety on him, because he cares for you.
—1 Pet. 5:6–7

God is with us in the midst of our fears, and He is in control over all that happens within our bodies. Let's look at some examples from Joshua and Psalm 139.

Have I not commanded you? Be strong and courageous.
Do not be frightened, and do not be dismayed, for the
LORD your God is with you wherever you go.
—Josh. 1:9

Where shall I go from your Spirit? Or where shall I
flee from your presence? If I ascend to heaven, you are
there! If I make my bed in Sheol, you are there! If I take
the wings of the morning and dwell in the uttermost
parts of the sea, even there your hand shall lead me,
and your right hand shall hold me. If I say, "Surely
the darkness shall cover me, and the light about me be
night," even the darkness is not dark to you; the night
is bright as the day, for darkness is as light with you.
—Ps. 139:7–12

God wasn't surprised when Sarah or I received news of our diagnoses. And He won't be caught off guard if the cancer returns. He walked with us once; He'll walk with us always.

Talking with friends or family is crucial. They walked with you through your treatments or surgeries. They'll walk with you through your fears. Many friends or family may not even realize you're struggling with fear of recurrence. Those who have never walked through cancer might assume you've returned to normal now that you're well. Say something to them such as "Sometimes I worry about my cancer coming back and what might happen if it does." Allow them to sit with this news for a few minutes, and don't expect them to tell you the cancer won't return. No one can predict the future, not even your oncologist.

My therapist and Sarah both have suggested talking with friends, family, and even yourself about *what is* instead of *what if.* Thoughts of *what if* leave things to chance and allow your mind to go to places that only seek to exacerbate the intensity of your fear. Focusing on *what is* allows your mind to concentrate on what is true. So what do you know to be true about your situation as it stands right this minute? Unless your doctor has told you otherwise, you know you don't have cancer. There is no proof that your cancer has returned, only a slight suspicion or fear that it has returned. The Apostle Paul wrote in Philippians 4:8, "Finally, brothers, whatever is true, whatever is honorable, whatever is just, whatever is pure, whatever is lovely, whatever is commendable, if there is any excellence, if there is anything worthy of praise, think about these things."

Your *what is* should include thinking about what is true, noble, honorable (or right), and more. Think about those things instead of the *what ifs* in your mind.

Talk with a professional therapist if the fear of recurrence overwhelms you. If you're not finding the help or support you need from family or friends, there is nothing wrong with seeking professional help. Ask for a referral to a therapist who works with other cancer survivors. My therapist spent nearly 15 years working in palliative care for cancer patients. She is the perfect fit for me to help me through the various emotions of navigating life after cancer, and I'm so grateful for her help and support.

Another thing Sarah recommends is not using Google as your source for information. "I don't google," she says. "It makes it worse for me if I go there." While the Internet is a fabulous place for information, it can also lead you down a rabbit hole of misinformation that leads to even greater fears than you could have imagined. Some information might be outdated or simply wrong. If you do feel the urge to google something, use reliable sources and make sure it's the most up-to-date information available. Also double-check your sources with other reliable sources, including asking your medical team. Begin with your nurse navigator if you have one. They are terrific at providing the latest information, statistics, data, and other news.

Finding ways to reduce stress can help alleviate the fear of recurrence. Spend time with family and friends without talking about cancer (unless you just need to talk about it). Focus on hobbies and other enjoyable activities such as listening to music or going for walks. Read a funny book or watch a funny show.

Make healthy choices for yourself. Eat nutritious meals and exercise regularly. Avoid unhealthy habits such as smoking, excessive drinking, or using drugs.

Be sure to follow your after-cancer care plan and allow yourself to be well-informed by your oncologist. If you're interested in knowing and don't know yet, find out what the chances of cancer returning are for you based on your type of cancer and your medical history. But keep in mind that your oncologist is simply sharing statistics, not predicting your future.

Finally, praying through scripture verses specifically focused on fear can help combat the fear of recurrence from occurring in the first place. One of my favorite verses when I struggle with the fear of recurrence is Isaiah 41:10: "Fear not, for I am with you; be not dismayed, for I am your God; I will strengthen you, I will help you, I will uphold you with my righteous right hand."

Going to God first will make all the difference in the world. Don't wait to go to Him. Too often, we allow ourselves to wallow in our emotions or talk to others for "expert" advice without first going to God with our concerns. This usually makes things worse because we are focused on the possibilities instead of what we know to be true of ourselves and of God. If God tells me not to be afraid, I know I don't have to be afraid. That doesn't mean the fears won't come. But I can take comfort in knowing He is with me in the midst of them and that He will uphold me through the fears. Trust in what is true, and God's Word is always true and trustworthy. And remember to think on these things.

Deeper Still ...

1. For cancer patients who are in remission, fear of recurrence is very common. Have you or someone you know struggled with this fear? If so, what were the triggers that brought the fear?

2. Has the fear of recurrence caused you to feel stuck and not able to return to a full normal life? What did you learn from this chapter that might be helpful?

3. Consider the list of ways to cope with fears of recurrence provided in this chapter.
   - Don't ignore your fears.
   - Focus on the facts.
   - Talk about what you're feeling.
   - Take it to God, praying and giving your fears to the Lord.

   Which of these do you think might be most helpful to you, and how do you plan to put them into practice?

4. Explain the difference between the *what is* and the *what if* described in this chapter.

5. What did you learn concerning ways to reduce stress and alleviate the fear of recurrence? Have you personally found other ways that are helpful?

6. Write out the words of the Apostle Paul in Philippians 4:8. It would be good to commit it to memory—helpful when you experience the fear of recurrence.

Chapter 5

CANCER GHOSTING: WHEN FRIENDS AND FAMILY LEAVE

The Word of God tells us in Ecclesiastes 3:1-2 (BSB), "To everything there is a season, and a time for every purpose under heaven: a time to be born and a time to die, a time to plant and a time to uproot." It is easy to take comfort in these words during difficult times. We know that not everything lasts forever, including challenging seasons in life. And sadly, that is true of relationships as well. Some people come into our lives for only a season. Some stay for a lifetime. And it's often in seasons of challenge when you find out who will be the ones to stay for a lifetime.

When you're faced with a cancer diagnosis, you fully expect those who have been there in years gone by to be there for the long haul. Unfortunately, many cancer patients find themselves the victim when friends and family members ghost them.

Cancer ghosting is a phenomenon when people literally disappear out of your life without word or warning and seemingly for no reason at all after your cancer diagnosis. One study found that 65 percent of respondents to a survey reported that they experienced cancer ghosting. That seems rather counterintuitive when it should be a time when friends and family come together to provide a cocoon of support.

Natasha Carlson wrote in her article "Cancer Ghosting Is an Unfortunate Reality" that she experienced this phenomenon from two dear friends, one whom she had shared a close relationship with for 22 years. "We had been through good times and bad times together, as is typical with a friendship that spans decades," she wrote. "But after I shared my diagnosis, I was very surprised to find that all contact with me was cut off. No responses to emails, texts, phone calls. Even when I was reaching out because I was confused and hurt, this did not generate any sort of reciprocal response."[7]

Being ghosted can be devastating, adding to the burden of the side effects of treatment, surgeries, and many other aspects of an already difficult journey. I had my own encounters with cancer ghosting. When I received my diagnosis, I directly contacted some family, friends, and members of our small group who had been praying for me after my biopsy. My husband contacted others, mostly by text since it was difficult to reach out to everyone. I was exhausted from the emotion of the day and retelling the diagnosis over and over. Our phones exploded with responses from so many people—except a few who surprised us with their silence.

As I write this, I've been cancer-free for more than three years, and I still haven't heard from those people. I've seen them at times when we happened to attend the same events. But in those moments, they never once asked me how I was doing or if I even still had cancer. In truth, they didn't say much of anything to me other than a casual greeting. I was stunned. I still am. More than that, I am hurt—deeply.

A wise woman once told me that "unreal expectations cause disappointments." Was I expecting too much from these people? Maybe. But I don't think so.

So what's behind cancer ghosting? There are myriad reasons someone might ghost a cancer patient. Here are just a few examples:

- People may be unsure how to help you and worry about saying the wrong thing.
- Cancer is a distressing reminder of our own mortality, and it may be too much for them to face.
- People experiencing trauma themselves may feel unable to provide emotional support to anyone else.
- People have an idea what cancer looks like and are scared to witness you go through it.
- People may feel guilty for living a happy life while you are suffering.
- Some people are afraid that cancer is contagious.
- People may feel the need to protect themselves, especially when watching someone deal with metastatic cancer. They simply can't be in it for the long haul.

Kerry McAvoy, PhD, shared in his blog "Accept People Will Come and Go" that "if you want to know the truth about someone, watch what he or she does, and ignore what he or she says. Behavior never lies. Acquaintances, family members, and friends will reveal their real intentions. Those who love us will show up when life takes a nasty turn."[8]

The most common reaction to cancer ghosting is an initial feeling of anger. Don't quench what you are feeling. But also don't sin in the anger. Ephesians 4:25–27 says, "Therefore, having put away falsehood, let each one of you speak the truth with his neighbor, for we are members one of another. Be angry and do not sin; do not let the sun go down on your anger, and give no opportunity to the devil." And definitely don't retaliate against them.

One common piece of advice from many therapists on the issue of ghosting in general is to determine if the relationship means enough to you to salvage it. Scripture tells us that we should always try to reconcile when possible. It also tells us to first go to the person with our grievance before we harbor it in our heart. Matthew 18:15 says, "If your brother sins against you, go and tell him his fault, between you and him alone. If he listens to you, you have gained your brother."

This will allow them a chance to explain themselves. But perhaps the relationship is beyond repair and reconciliation isn't possible. Search your heart and seek God's face about reconciliation, but if you deem it isn't a reality, say goodbye in your own way. You can do that by writing a letter to that person without sending it. Tell them your questions and your pain. Tell them how their actions and inactions have wounded you. And tell them that it's time to part ways. Trust them to the Lord and release them into His care. You can either destroy the letter you write or keep it for yourself, but never send it to the person.

It's hard to give up on someone you're emotionally invested in, even if they have hurt you. If you need to walk away, give yourself permission to grieve the loss before moving on.

If you feel that the person is someone you want to put the energy into and salvage the relationship, reach out once more (if you haven't done so already). If you do decide to make one last ditch effort to salvage that relationship, keep in mind that they might not respond. Is that a risk you're willing to take? Figure out how to have a conversation with them if they do respond. When you are finally able to have that conversation, speak truth to them in love and grace. Use "I" statements instead of accusatory "you" statements. Ask questions. And let them share without interruption.

If you have reached out but they don't respond, stop attempting to reach out. A nonresponse is an indication that you're being ghosted, and they're not interested in reconciling. If the person does decide to respond, accepts your invitation to have a conversation, and wants to renew the relationship, keep in mind that it's okay to set boundaries in that renewed relationship. Remember that 1 Corinthians 13:4–6 says, "Love is patient and kind; love does not envy or boast; it is not arrogant or rude. It does not insist on its own way; it is not irritable or resentful; it does not rejoice at wrongdoing, but rejoices with the truth."

Lysa TerKeurst in her book *Good Boundaries and Goodbyes* explains that boundaries are actually a positive aspect to relationship dynamics. "We set boundaries so we know what to do when we very much want to love those around us really well without losing ourselves in the process. Good boundaries help us preserve the love within us even when some relationships become unsustainable and we must accept the reality of a goodbye."⁹

When asked about the greatest commandment in the Law, Jesus replied to the Pharisee, "You shall love the Lord your God with all your heart and with all your soul and with all your mind. This is the great and first commandment. And a second is like it: You shall love your neighbor as yourself" (Matt. 22:37–39).

So how do we love our neighbor as ourselves? Jesus loves us unconditionally, and that should be our posture with others as well. We should treat others the way we want to be treated, and we should treat them with kindness and respect, not expecting anything in return.

If that's true, why wasn't I—the one ghosted—loved in this way? We have to see that ghosting isn't an act of love but rather a dysfunction. As TerKeurst says, "But we can't enable bad behavior in ourselves and others and call it love. We can't tolerate destructive patterns and call it love."¹⁰

Too often Christians have the idea that being a Christian requires us to believe the best about others no matter what. But that is an unhealthy attitude when it comes to establishing boundaries. It is not unchristian to require people to treat you in healthy ways.

God is the author of boundaries. For example, He determined at the creation of the world that there would be boundaries among the waters and the sky.

Do you not fear me? declares the LORD. Do you not tremble before me? I placed the sand as the boundary for the sea, a perpetual barrier that it cannot pass;

> *though the waves toss, they cannot prevail; though*
> *they roar, they cannot pass over it.*
>
> —Jer. 5:22

God would place boundaries between man and beast and birds. There would be boundaries in the Garden of Eden. In Genesis 2, we see how God set up boundaries for Adam and Eve. But it wasn't for their detriment. It was for their freedom.

> *And the Lord God commanded the man, saying, "You*
> *may surely eat of every tree of the garden, but of the tree*
> *of the knowledge of good and evil you shall not eat, for*
> *in the day that you eat of it you shall surely die."*
>
> —Gen. 2:16–17

He didn't place these boundaries on them because he was trying to be cruel. He knew that the consequences of disobeying the boundaries would mean death for the ones He created and loved. And as we know, our first parents did disobey, and we are all suffering the consequences of those actions today.

Setting boundaries in family relationships or friendships is for the betterment of both parties. As TerKeurst explained in her book, "Love can be unconditional but relational access never should be. God loves us but He has established that sin causes separation from Him. When Adam and Eve sinned, they were no longer given the same kind of access."[11] Thankfully, we have a Savior in Jesus Christ who has provided us a way back to the Father through the spilled blood on the cross at Calvary.

In setting up boundaries, however, don't do so out of bitterness or spite. Ephesians 4:31–32 reminds us, "Let all bitterness and wrath and anger and clamor and slander be put away from you, along with all malice. Be kind to one another, tender-hearted, forgiving one another, as God in Christ forgave you."

Examine your own heart and make sure you're setting healthy boundaries for you and the other person, and that you're not simply making a list of get-even demands. Trust may be hard to rebuild, so set those boundaries and start at a pace you're comfortable with.

Regardless of what happens with your relationship—broken or healed—at some point, you must find a way to forgive them. Matthew 6:14–15 tells us, "For if you forgive others their trespasses, your heavenly Father will also forgive you, but if you do not forgive others their trespasses, neither will your Father forgive your trespasses."

You may be angry. You may be experiencing grief and sadness at this loss. There may be a sense of confusion at the way you've been treated. No matter what you're feeling, you need to forgive, even if the person who wronged you never asks for it.

Another way to help you grieve the loss of a relationship through ghosting is to focus on the people God has put in your life. How has your circle of friends been there for you? Did you receive meals, cards, flowers, prayers, and text messages from others? Focus on those connections that never left you. Consider sending thank you notes to encourage those who have been encouraging you. If you don't have a circle of friends yet, find one in your local church or through cancer support groups in your community, but always keep boundaries in the back of your mind.

Romans 12:18 says, "If possible, so far as it depends on you, live peaceably with all." Read that again. If possible. So far as it depends on you. You can try for reconciliation as described above and even establish clear boundaries for moving forward in the relationship, but sometimes reconciliation isn't possible. And sometimes it's not up to you. You must accept the goodbye and move forward.

If you do decide to close the door on a relationship, try to change the narrative in your own mind from "they don't care about me" to "perhaps they are unable to provide me what I need from a relationship." That could help you find closure when ending that relationship.

While cancer ghosting can be hurtful, it is important to remember that it is not a reflection of the person with cancer. It says more about the other person's fears and emotions surrounding themselves and cancer. It is important for those going through cancer who have been ghosted to seek out support from others who are willing and able to be there for them during their treatment journey.

I still don't know the reason for the ghosting I experienced. For now, I have determined that I don't want to know their excuses. And while I would welcome the opportunity to reconcile with them, I'm trying to figure out what that would look like for me with boundaries established before moving ahead is even possible. Trust that taking time in this process is going to be beneficial to your own mental and spiritual health. I have forgiven all of them, and I'm not bitter as I was when it initially happened. Keeping an intentional distance is what my soul needs at the moment.

Right now my focus and attention isn't on the ones who left me. I am finding ways to remind myself of the amazing community that God surrounded me with during my cancer treatment and surgeries. I was so blessed with the hands and feet of Jesus from hundreds—and I mean literally hundreds—of people. Yes, it hurt to be ghosted, but I serve a sovereign God who was not taken by surprise by their actions. He knew this would happen, and He was in it with me when it happened. He provided me with beautiful relationships in ways I never imagined was possible when I received my diagnosis. The faithfulness of God—I can trust in that, and so can you.

All of this is normal and healthy as you consider your own path forward from cancer ghosting. Pray and trust God to work out the details whether it is a relationship with boundaries or a goodbye.

Deeper Still …

1. As you read this chapter, perhaps *cancer ghosting* was a new term to you. If you have experienced cancer ghosting during your cancer journey, how did it make you feel? Be specific and honest with your answer using words that best describe how you felt.

2. Is there someone—a friend or family member—who disappeared at a time when you needed them most? Pray, asking the Lord to reveal anyone to you that you may need to reach out to or even forgive. Ask for Him to provide you with the wisdom and discernment to know how to respond.

3. How has my own personal story of experiencing cancer ghosting been an encouragement to you by providing helpful suggestions for how to respond?

4. Jesus was abandoned by His closest companions as He went to the cross. He understands your pain and wants to be invited into your deepest hurts. Jesus promised us, "I will never leave you nor forsake you." What comfort and assurance does this bring you?

5. This chapter helps explain the concept of boundaries. Record all you learned and perhaps something you plan to implement in your own life.

Chapter 6

INTIMACY IN MARRIAGE AFTER CANCER TREATMENT

Mark and Hannah (not their real names) are now empty nesters in their late 50s. Their children are away from home, one working in insurance and the other serving his country in the Armed Forces. While they missed their son and daughter, they were enjoying this new phase in life when their time was their own again. By Hannah's account, they were even enjoying a more romantic life since the kids were out of the house. They found themselves relishing in activities together as well as a physical intimacy that enhanced their marital relationship.

But then everything changed. Hannah had been faithful to get yearly mammograms since she turned 40. She had rather dense breast tissue, which made seeing the images from the mammograms difficult and requiring an ultrasound at times if there was something concerning. So she didn't think it odd when a nurse from the breast center called and said they wanted to do an ultrasound on something they found in the imaging of her left breast.

Hannah reported for the ultrasound two days later. She waited, lying on a stiff table in a dimly lit room for the technician to return to tell her it was nothing. However, the technician had other news for her. She reported to Hannah that the radiologist discovered what looked like a cyst but couldn't say with exact certainty that it was benign. He recommended that Hannah get a biopsy.

Hannah immediately panicked. So many questions ran through her mind. *Will the biopsy hurt? What if it's cancer? Why would I have cancer? I don't have a history of cancer in my family. How do I tell Mark and my kids? They'll fall apart if it's cancer.*

The technician tried to calm her fears. She told Hannah the biopsy shouldn't hurt, and it was a quick procedure. While the technician did her best to allay Hannah's fears, Hannah left the breast center a ball of nerves. She was in tears and called Mark from the car. Mark lovingly reassured Hannah that she would be okay, and they would walk together through whatever was to come. Six days later, Hannah was diagnosed with stage 2 triple-negative cancer. She would face months of grueling chemotherapy and a bilateral mastectomy. She opted for reconstruction after the mastectomy.

"We were still young," explained Hannah who is now five years removed from her cancer diagnosis. "We were still enjoying each other physically. I felt like having breasts would continue to be an important part of enhancing intimacy in our marriage.

And I wanted to still feel feminine. I wanted that for him as much as I wanted it for me."

However, the reconstruction with implants left Hannah feeling anything but sexy or desirable. Her new breasts had scars across the middle of them from the mastectomy, and she was left without nipples. She had very little sensation in her breasts, especially along the scar lines that continued down her sides almost to her back where they had to remove some excess skin during reconstruction.

"I felt like I looked like someone had taken an axe to my chest and left me horribly disfigured," Hannah said. "I was happy with the implants themselves, but I hated the way I looked because of the scars."

Hannah says it was difficult for her to find energy and strength for intimacy with Mark during her chemo treatments. She thought all of that would change once the surgeries were behind her. But things only got worse. She hadn't anticipated how she would feel with the scars on her breasts. So she often rebuffed Mark's attempts at intimacy, not ever giving him a reason why she "wasn't in the mood."

"I couldn't stand looking at myself in the mirror," she said. "I found myself repulsive, and if I felt that way, I knew Mark would feel the same way."

Hannah says she "caved" a few times but always left on her bra. Mark groaned about the bra but always relented when he saw that she was more comfortable wearing it.

In the meantime, Mark was left wondering what was wrong with his wife. "She'd struggled with some body image issues before cancer, which everyone does to some degree," Mark said.

"But I thought we'd worked through those. Besides, this was a severe reversal to what we'd been experiencing after the last kid left the house."

Mark said wearing the bra during sex was the last straw. He'd dealt with Hannah's rejections for months, and although he always asked why she wasn't in the mood, she deferred. "She blamed her lack of interest on lingering effects of chemo," said Mark. "But when this went on for months and months, I knew something else was going on."

And there *was* something else going on. Hannah was experiencing deeper body image issues—issues that she never imagined would impact her in such a dramatic fashion. And she was unwilling to talk to Mark about her feelings. She was afraid he would dismiss her thoughts and feelings as being silly.

Mark, frustrated and confused, encouraged Hannah to visit with a counselor about the issues that were plaguing their sex life. He tried to get her to understand that whatever she was feeling about intimacy after cancer is likely normal.

In fact, it is quite normal for both men and women to struggle in the intimacy department after cancer and cancer surgeries. According to one poll conducted by LiveStrong, nearly 60 percent of all cancer survivors reported experiencing sexual dysfunction after treatment. As many as 85 to 90 percent of survivors of prostate, breast, and gynecologic cancer reported long-term concerns regarding physical intimacy. Post-cancer sexual concerns may be both mental and physical in nature. And that impacts both the survivor and the spouse. A survivor's spouse may be worried about emotionally pressuring or causing physical pain. A survivor may feel nervous about how their spouse will respond to changes in their physical appearance.

Stephanie Ross, PhD, a clinical health psychologist and founder and director of Illness Navigation Resources, said in a recent podcast on the topic of tips for talking to a spouse about sex after cancer that the basis for great sex is communication. "Your sex life may become medicalized as patient and caregiver," she said. "You need to return to being partners, and that doesn't happen without communication."

Ross suggests recreating the bond and building the bond you had before cancer through some nonsexual activities. "Commit to 30 minutes of alone time without sex," she said. "Watch a show, exercise, go for a walk, cuddle in a nonsexual way."

Ross said it can be difficult to have conversations about such an intimate and sometimes embarrassing subject. "Have a series of conversations," she recommends. "Reconnect and work your way up to the details of what you want to talk about." Ross insisted that it doesn't all have to spill out in one conversation.

Some intimacy issues after cancer treatment or surgery are emotional (such as body image), while other issues are functional—and neither of them is wrong. There are multiple side effects that men and women experience during and after treatment and surgeries for cancer. For example, women might experience early menopause, loss of libido, loss of sexual function or sensation, fatigue, or even anxiety, depression, or fear.

Cancer treatments often cause changes to men's sexual function as well. For example, pelvic radiation or surgery for prostate or other cancers may impact a man's ability to get or maintain an erection. Hormone therapy that lowers testosterone levels may impact sex drive. Treatments such as chemotherapy or radiation therapy may cause nausea, lethargy, or pain, which diminishes sex drive. Other side effects may include an inability to reach orgasm or for men to ejaculate.

While it can be embarrassing to talk about issues such as disfigured breasts, vaginal dryness, or erectile dysfunction, Ross said that couples should "work on ways to acknowledge that the body is not the enemy. Recognize that it is different and work with what is or isn't there any longer. There should never be shame associated with sex after cancer surgery."

Hannah did eventually go to counseling. Her therapist helped her acknowledge that she was grieving the loss of her breasts, something that once made her feel feminine. She also admitted that her new breasts didn't feel real, so she didn't feel as feminine as she once did. She worried if her breasts didn't feel real to her, what would Mark feel when he touched her?

Hannah said she also knows that men are attracted and often aroused by what they see. She worried that Mark wouldn't find her breasts attractive anymore. A default in many relationships is for the spouse to say, "I love your body anyway." This can be a turnoff to many cancer survivors. That was true for Hannah and Mark. "It felt like something he had to say because he's my husband," Hannah said. "I just didn't believe it was true."

Mark had to work hard to get Hannah to believe their love was deeper than what he saw in her appearance. His love extended beyond the physical, so their physical relationship was deeper than that. It was deeply personal and soul-fulfilling, and because it was ordained by God, it was a blessing to be able to be physical with her at all.

Josh Squires, Pastor of Counseling and Congregational Care at First Presbyterian Church in Columbia, South Carolina, wrote an article in 2016 called, "Marital Intimacy Is More Than Sex." He said that intimacy is a multifaceted thing, and there are five types of intimacy.

The first and most foundational type of intimacy is spiritual intimacy. "Spiritual intimacy can be seen as the hub from which all other intimacy types protrude," Squires wrote. "If spiritual intimacy is high, then the other types of intimacy, though they will have seasons of greater or lesser intensity, will have a certain level of natural resiliency." He explained that spiritual intimacy comes from being in the Word together, praying for one another and worshiping together. "When we are on the same spiritual diet, we can expect to grow in similar ways and therefore grow together—not separately."[12]

Next is recreational intimacy, the bond that is created and strengthened by doing activities together. "This sort of intimacy tends to be its highest early in the relationship when both partners are willing to do and try things outside of their comfort zone just to have the opportunity to be in each other's presence," said Squires.[13] However, as life gets more complicated with responsibilities, engaging in recreational intimacy becomes more challenging. Nonetheless, God has made us to enjoy life's activities with our spouses.

Third is intellectual intimacy, the activity of connecting to one another by discussing certain issues such as politics or like-minded interests. Like recreational intimacy, this tends to be heightened at the beginning of a relationship when you're getting to know one another.

Fourth is physical intimacy, the domain most people think of when they hear the word *intimate*. "This includes but is not limited to sexual activity," said Squires. "There is also non-sexual physical intimacy such as holding hands, cuddling on the couch, or a hug."[14]

Finally, there is emotional intimacy, the sharing of your own experiences with another. "Men are called to shepherd their wife's heart just as much as women are called to shepherd their husband's sexuality," Squires explained. "Just as men feel most connected when physical intimacy is highest, women generally feel most connected when emotional intimacy is highest."[15]

Squires suggested that there are cycles of intimacy and cycles of isolation within the context of marriage. When men feel disconnected, they often try to get physical with their wife. When women feels disconnected, they often try to engage their husband in emotional intimacy. "Both spouses feel the disconnection but are trying to resolve the problem in opposite ways," he said. "Here couples can easily find themselves in cycles of isolation. ... This is where the Christian commitment to love one another, even when it hurts, ... can help the couple move from cycles of isolation to cycles of intimacy as they lovingly put each other's needs before their own."[16]

Here are some scripture examples of the Christian commitment to love one another.

- John 13:34–35: "A new commandment I give to you, that you love one another: just as I have loved you, you also are to love one another. By this all people will know that you are my disciples, if you have love for one another."

- Galatians 5:13: "For you were called to freedom, brothers. Only do not use your freedom as an opportunity for the flesh, but through love serve one another."
- Ephesians 4:2 "With all humility and gentleness, with patience, bearing with one another in love."

Squires recommends that couples pray about sex. More specifically, they should pray for desire, for the removal of distractions, and for delight. Once you have prayed, talk about sex with your spouse and then simply have sex. While it's easy to say to simply have sex, sometimes it isn't so simple when you're faced with the devasting effects of cancer treatments and surgery. But when we leave our physical relationship with our spouse in the hands of the One who created physical intimacy, we might be surprised at what He will do.

Hannah noted that her therapist suggested she take the time to take care of herself. Often, we are too busy meeting the needs of others and forget what we need for ourselves. Regarding Hannah's body image issues, her therapist suggested rebuilding her self-image. Hannah pointed out that she had to give herself time to adjust.

"It takes time to process and accept a cancer diagnosis, and it's life-changing," she said. "I had to give myself time to adjust to a new way of feeling about my body and the way I look now. I had to find ways to appreciate and respect new things about my body and to acknowledge the difficult journey my body has been through."

Hannah said it also took time for her to adjust to her new breasts—the way they feel, the way they look, the scars, the lack of sensation. All of it required a period of adjustment before she felt comfortable again.

It took a couple of years for Hannah to break through her body image insecurities and fully trust her body with Mark again. Once she was able to open up to her therapist about her body image issues, she found it easier to share her feelings with Mark. "I just told Mark what I told the therapist," said Hannah. "But the first step was opening the lines of communication with him. I had to be able to trust him with my heart before I could trust him with my body."

Hannah still doesn't relish the idea of scars on her breasts, but she is learning to love the body that she has because it is the one God designed for her for such a time as this. Mark was happy to attend some therapy sessions with Hannah as well as individually to learn how he could be most helpful and supportive of her while she worked through these difficult issues. Together, they are much more secure in their physical connection and have returned to having an enjoyable physical relationship in their marriage.

"It isn't perfect, and I don't always feel attractive or desirable," explained Hannah. "But I am learning to trust that Mark's love for me is deeper than the physical, and that's a beautiful thing."

Deeper Still ...

1. Surgery from having cancer often brings body image issues. These should never be dismissed but talked about. The effects can be both mental and physical, emotional and functional. If you've been suffering with body image issues, have you shared with someone (a therapist, a friend, or your spouse) your thoughts and feelings?

2. Communication is key in any marriage relationship but especially when related to sex after cancer surgeries. If the subject of sexual intimacy is difficult for you and your spouse to talk about, what nonsexual activities can you enjoy together?

3. Both emotional and physical intimacy are gifts from God and ones to be enjoyed. From the five types of intimacy mentioned in this chapter, which one (or ones) could you spend time working on to better your marriage relationship?

4. In your experience with having sex after cancer surgery, have you felt embarrassed, ashamed, or unattractive? If so, how have you responded to those feelings?

5. Sexual intimacy is not only physical but spiritual as well. Do you currently spend time praying about sex? If not, God invites you to pray for this gift He has given you and your spouse. Remember, when we leave our physical relationship with our spouse in the hands of the One who created physical intimacy, we might be surprised at what He will do.

Chapter 7

FINDING JOY IN SUFFERING

If all you did was listen to the news, you'd assume there is absolutely no joy in this world. It often feels like the weight of this world has no end. And that's without considering the misery some of our family and friends might be experiencing. So maybe there's some truth to part of my opening sentence—there is absolutely no joy in this world.

But what exactly does it mean to have joy? Happiness and joy aren't the same thing. Happiness is mostly dependent on external circumstances and rarely lasts for extended periods of time. In fact, Merriam-Webster defines *happy* as "fortunate, glad, or pleased." All those things are fleeting. Joy, on the other hand, is something that is manifest deep within ourselves and is rarely dependent on circumstances or events. Merriam-Webster defines it as "an emotion evoked by well-being." A dear friend described it best when she said joy is the "deep-seated confidence in the sovereignty of God." There is also an element of surrender in joy—surrendering it all to Him and basking in the knowledge that He is in complete control.

Taking all of that into consideration, I want to suggest that there is indeed joy in this world. In fact, there is joy in the midst of suffering. How is that possible? Does it make sense that joy comes only in the absence of suffering? Or perhaps joy comes after suffering. The Bible tells us that joy does come after suffering and is also present in the middle of our suffering. I can say that because I have experienced both firsthand.

I remember vividly when I received my cancer diagnosis that the negative person in me immediately went to, well, the negative. I just expected that the entirety of my treatments would be filled with misery, suffering, pain, fatigue, and vomiting, and would be devoid of any type of joy whatsoever. What I found, however, was the exact opposite. What I discovered instead was a joy that I had never known before.

Yes, there was a lot of suffering in the form of pain, fatigue, nausea, loss, and so much more. But God introduced me to joy that came in the form of His people and His presence. As I shared in my story from Part I, I learned of my diagnosis when I was in a leaders' meeting for our church's women's Bible study. Those women surrounded me with literal and figurative hugs from that very moment of diagnosis and continued to keep me surrounded throughout my chemo treatments and subsequent surgeries. They practically demanded updates on how I was doing—fears as well as triumphs—and they prayed. Oh, how they prayed over me fervently and faithfully. They showered me with indescribable joy.

Remember the meals those people brought us? They were delicious and wonderful, and so were the few minutes they spent with me when they dropped them off. It brought me such joy to see the joy that it brought them to be able to serve me and my family so graciously.

And the visitors who came every other week—how I loved to see them. On the days when it wasn't too hot, my guests and I sat outside on the porch and just talked. Sometimes we talked about my cancer journey. Other times we talked about everything else under the sun. Usually there was the gift of a sweet, iced tea for me, which always brought a smile to my face. Many brought gifts or cards. The joy of those visits made my suffering tolerable and manageable. I was always exhausted when they left, but I also always had a grin from ear to ear and was so excited for the next day's visitor. Those visits carried me through some dark, dark days, and I will be eternally grateful for them. They brought me joy in the midst of my suffering.

Yes, I found joy in things, people, and circumstances. But what about God? I found great joy in Him as well. There was joy in His presence. I found it when I prayed, which I admit wasn't as often as I would have liked. I struggled with praying on most days. It wasn't that I was angry, hurt, sad, or any other emotion you can insert here. I honestly didn't know what to say to God. I asked Him to heal me and help control the pain and nausea. I asked Him to bless Kurt and my mom as they cared for me. I always thanked Him for the people who served us so graciously. But they weren't the deep prayers I had anticipated. Sometimes all I had the strength to mutter was "heal me." I know He heard me. And I know He was always with me. I felt His presence daily, moment by moment. Psalm 16:11 says, "You make known to me the path of life; in your presence there is fullness of joy; at your right hand are pleasures forevermore." I felt that deeply, and in it was joy.

As a cancer patient, you can't help but be faced with your own mortality. I stared death in the face, and yes, it frightened me. But I knew that if God chose to heal me by taking me home, I was safe and satisfied in the knowledge of where I was going. It's not exactly a pleasant thought to have, but it brought me great joy in remembering my salvation. Psalm 20:5 says, "May we shout for joy over your salvation, and in the name of our God set up our banners!"

In being forced to look at eternity, I was reminded of the joy in His glory and in my future glory. Romans 8:17 says, "And if [we are] children, then heirs—heirs of God and fellow heirs with Christ, provided we suffer with him in order that we may also be glorified with him." How can we not find joy in the midst of our suffering when we focus on the One (Jesus) who suffered for us?

Timothy Keller in his book *Walking with God Through Pain and Suffering* reminds us of the *why* of our suffering and our ultimate joy. He said this in reference to Jesus:

> The sovereign God himself has come down into this world and has experienced its darkness. He has personally drunk the cup of its suffering down to the dregs. And he did it not to justify himself but to justify us, that is, to bear the suffering, death, and curse for sin that we have earned. He takes the punishment upon himself so that someday he can return and end all evil without having to condemn and punish us.[17]

Isn't that reason enough to be joyful, even in the midst of suffering? Yet many still ask why? Why must we suffer? God has a purpose in all things in our lives, including our suffering. He uses our suffering for His glory and our good. Keller, who himself died of pancreatic cancer in 2023, unpacked this further in his book.

> First, suffering transforms our attitude toward ourselves. It humbles us and removes unrealistic self-regard and pride. It shows us how fragile we are… Second, suffering will profoundly change our relationship to the good things in our lives. We will see that some things have become too important to us.

> Keller went on to say, "Suffering can strengthen our relationship to God as nothing else can. Finally, suffering is almost a prerequisite if we are going to be of much use to other people, especially when they go through their own trials. Adversity makes us far more compassionate than we could have been otherwise."[18]

So how can joy come in our sorrow? Theologian John Piper spoke on this topic in a sermon in 2021 and shared from 2 Corinthians 6:10, which says we are "sorrowful, yet always rejoicing." He posits that joy follows sorrow, and there is joy in our sorrow. And of course, Piper backs it up with texts from the Word of God.

Where joy follows sorrow, Psalm 30:5 tells us, "For his [God's] anger is but for a moment, and his favor is for a lifetime. Weeping may tarry for the night, but joy comes with the morning." According to Piper, when the psalmist wrote this, he meant tearful joy in God will be "replaced with tearless joy in God. Painful joy in God will be replaced with painless joy in God."

Jesus spoke to His disciples about what it would be like to see Him die and then live again.

> *Truly, truly I say to you, you will weep and lament, but the world will rejoice. You will be sorrowful, but your sorrow will turn into joy. When a woman is giving birth, she has sorrow because her hour has come, but when she has delivered the baby, she no longer remembers the anguish, for joy that a human being has been born into this world. So also you have sorrow now, but I will see you again, and your hearts will rejoice, and no one will take your joy from you*
> *—John 16:20–22*

Piper also pointed out the joy that comes *in* sorrow. Philippians 4:4 tells us, "Rejoice in the Lord always; again I will say, rejoice." That means we can and should rejoice, even in the midst of our suffering. We don't necessarily rejoice *for* our suffering, but *in* it.

> *We rejoice in our sufferings, knowing that suffering produces endurance, and endurance produces character, and character produces hope, and hope does not put us to shame, because God's love has been poured into our hearts through the Holy Spirit who has been given to us.*
> *—Rom. 5:3–5*

Eric Bobbitt at Zionsville Fellowship said it this way about those who have had cancer and suffered greatly with the disease: "There is a joy to be experienced in suffering. There's a joy that comes and there's a depth that comes with suffering. I find that people who have suffered are more gentle; they're more empathetic, and there's just a calm about them that people who haven't had cancer don't have."

Bob Ash at Zionsville Fellowship agreed:

> We're not getting nailed to a cross, but we're getting a glimpse of what suffering is. Let's embrace the suffering for a while and say, "How can that suffering bring us more joy?" Well, can we start looking at how we're learning more about Christ? If that brings me closer to Jesus, and somebody can see that in me, and that gives them a shot at eternity that they wouldn't have had otherwise, you bet it's worth it.

And we can count it all joy when we suffer. In fact, James 1:2-4 tells us. "Count it all joy, my brothers, when you meet trials of various kinds, for you know that the testing of your faith produces steadfastness. And let steadfastness have its full effect, that you may be perfect and complete, lacking in nothing."

"Count it all joy" isn't simply a suggestion; it's a command. But we recognize that in any trial there is loss, and you have to find joy in the mist of loss and grief. We can see that there is a natural progression. Testing leads to steadfastness, which leads to completeness. Completeness is the goal for which Christ saved us.

Ash also said, "God didn't come into the world to save us from suffering. He didn't come into the world to save us from cancer. He came into the world to save us from our sins. He came into the world so we wouldn't have to suffer an eternity in hell."

We are sorrowful yet always rejoicing. So how in the world do we endure the suffering to experience the joy?

- We know that we can endure suffering because God will use it for our good and for His glory. He will teach us through it and make us more like Jesus in the process.
- We know we can endure suffering because God will eventually end our suffering. There is an end to all our suffering. There is a time limit on our suffering. That may happen here on earth in some period of time, or it may end in heaven if He calls us home. Or it may end when Jesus returns. Whichever way it happens, suffering will end.
- We know we can endure suffering because God will reveal Himself to us in our suffering. God will speak to us through His Spirit to reveal His great love and compassion for us in our suffering.
- We know that we can endure suffering because God will receive our suffering, our lamentations, our cries, our pleas, and our grief. He will receive all of them.

There is a steadfastness in suffering and finding joy in the midst of it. Steadfastness in the face of suffering and sorrow means to tenaciously withstand a trial until God removes it at His appointed time. But there is also lamenting when we suffer, which can lead to joy. Lamenting holds joy's hand and is the pathway to joy.

How do we start to find joy in the midst of suffering? A dear friend shared this acronym with me:

J   Look to **Jesus** for His help first.
O   Concentrate on how you can serve **others.**
Y   Then take care of **yourself.**

It isn't easy to endure the trial of cancer, but we can trust that we aren't alone in our suffering, and in that, there is joy. Perhaps you are in the midst of your cancer journey and aren't feeling the joy that comes in the midst of suffering. Rest assured that joy will come if you put your faith in the One who brings true joy. We don't know the timing or plans of our Father in heaven, but we can count on this promise: "He will wipe away every tear from their eyes, and death shall be no more, neither shall there be mourning, nor crying, nor pain anymore, for the former things have passed away" (Rev. 21:4).

Deeper Still ...

1. From what you learned in this chapter, how would you describe the difference between happiness and joy?
2. The gift of the presence of other people can provide comfort in your time of suffering. During your time of treatment with cancer, how did you experience the comfort of others?
3. The Bible teaches us that God's presence can be experienced tangibly. When we draw near to Him, He promises to draw near to us. Explain how God's presence comforted you during your time of suffering.

AFTER CANCER: NOW WHAT?

4. It can be difficult to understand the purpose God has for our suffering. He asks us to trust Him and promises that our suffering will not be wasted but rather used for our good. How have you grown in the areas of humility, gratitude, compassion, and faith during your time of suffering?

5. What examples were given on how to endure the suffering in order to experience joy?

6. Do you have the hope that is available in Jesus and the promise of eternal life with Him where there will no longer be any suffering or pain or death? If not, talk to a Christian friend or pastor—or simply pray.

Chapter 8

THE HANDS AND FEET OF JESUS: WHY COMMUNITY AND FAITH MATTER

The day I rang the bell after my last chemo treatment was special for multiple reasons. Ringing the bell signifies (to many) that you're cancer free. For others, it's to mark the end of your chemotherapy or radiation therapy treatments. I hadn't gotten the last of my test results to know for certain I was cancer-free, so for me, ringing the bell marked the end of treatment. I was a bucket of tears when I rang the bell. But they were tears of joy. I was in such pain and felt tremendous fatigue and nausea, but I also felt like I could have run a marathon because of the excitement I had flowing through me. It brought me such happiness to not have to schedule my next chemo treatment. I checked out and left the building with a full and thankful heart.

Kurt, my mom, family, and friends were all there that day. I realized that community matters when it comes to healing from cancer or living with metastatic cancer. I remember someone saying to me after the bell-ringing ceremony and celebration that they were overjoyed that I had such a faithful community to help me through my darkest days. "I don't know how people do this without faith and without community," she said. I couldn't agree more.

I will never forget what all those people did for me during my time of suffering. If you know someone who has just been diagnosed with cancer or has been going through the journey for a period of time, check in with them. Send a text or call and ask them what they need most. Offer to visit them or pray for them, and then follow through with whatever they need. Don't fall into the trap of not being there for them. Everyone needs a community to surround them while going through cancer.

There's no rule book on what to do or say to someone who has been diagnosed with a potentially fatal disease. Here are some suggestions on things to say—and not say—in these circumstances.

What to Say to a Person with a Serious Illness

- "I don't know what to say, but please know how much I care." Be honest if you're at a loss for words. Don't fill your conversation with empty words or platitudes. If necessary, be quiet and simply listen.
- "What can I do for you?" Ask them genuinely and then give them what they've asked for, within reason.
- "I'm always here if you ever want to talk." If you say it, mean it, and then do it.
- "I'm so sorry this has happened to you."

What *Not* to Say to a Person with a Serious Illness

- "I know exactly how you feel." Unless you've experienced a cancer journey of your own, you don't know exactly how they feel, so don't pretend that you do. That can make the person feel that their situation isn't that big of a deal.

- "When (fill in the blank) had this, (fill in the blank) happened." Don't compare one person's story with someone else's. You may think you're being hopeful, but you never know how a person with a serious diagnosis is going to internalize your well-intentioned anecdotes.

- "You're so brave" or "You're so strong." You might think this is an encouraging thing to say, but it might actually put pressure on the person to act differently than they are feeling. While a person with a serious illness might be strong on certain days, most days they don't feel that way, and hearing this might be disheartening to them.

- "I'm sure you'll be fine." Telling a person with a serious illness they'll be fine or not to worry can be misconstrued as making light of their situation. It also promotes a false sense of certainty.

Other Things to Do and Not Do for a Person with a Serious Illness

- DO meet them where they are. If the person is struggling with their illness, don't approach them in an overly positive manner. Instead help them work toward acceptance.

- DON'T put them at fault. This is not the time to fault someone for their diagnosis. A person with lung cancer who smoked for years doesn't need to be criticized for their past decisions.
- DON'T make their diagnosis their identity. Cancer doesn't define you. How you deal with the disease is what defines you.
- DON'T treat them as helpless. Don't assume they want your help. Ask them what they need and then provide it.
- DO include them. Don't shun the one dealing with this disease. And don't assume they don't want to be included in activities just because they are ill.
- DO give them grace. Give grace in the context of what they're going through. They may not be in the best of spirits, and they may not act like the person you knew before their diagnosis.
- DO pray for them. It's just that simple. Pray. This is the greatest and best way you can help them.

Remember Sarah, the 37-year-old woman with breast cancer? She experienced the gift of community during her journey in 2023. "I don't think I've ever felt so much love and support in all my life," she said. "I know I have an awesome community. But the way they showed up, and then you think, 'Oh, everybody's showing up at the beginning.' But they didn't stop showing up!"

If you don't have a community to lean into during your cancer journey, talk to your medical team. There are many community cancer support centers throughout the United States (and beyond) that will provide you with resources to deal with your cancer journey, including counseling. Being together with others who are going through what you're dealing with is healing. There's a camaraderie you can't have with those who have never had cancer before. Everyone should have a community of friends, family, and even acquaintances to help them during their journey. It's scriptural to meet together with others, especially in a time of need. Hebrews 10:24–25 tells us, "Let us consider how to stir up one another to love and good works, not neglecting to meet together, as is the habit of some, but encouraging one another, and all the more as you see the Day drawing near."

The other thing that bolstered Sarah during her cancer journey was her faith in God. "I can't imagine doing this without my faith," Sarah said. "God is in control. He has a plan for me, and I'm not in this alone."

Sarah noted that for so long she would pray for God to take this away from her. But she realized that she needed to pray for Him to prepare her for whatever lies ahead. "I've been really trying to pray more for that, and to just help me prepare my steps for whatever the road looks like in front of me."

Eric Bobbitt said that cancer brings to the forefront and compresses the questions you need to ask about life. And for many of those questions, faith plays a vital role. "What's the meaning of suffering?" he asked. "It really brings the invisible to the forefront. Cancer is of the body, so it's actually a physical reality, but it brings the immaterial so much closer than regular life does."

He went on to say that you will find yourself asking questions such as "Is this all there is? What's behind life? What's behind the veil?" And suddenly you realize your mortality, realizing you might not be here as long as you thought you would be. "We all kind of wonder about that, but cancer forces you to deal with those things," Bobbitt said. "And then faith brings an understanding to all of that. There's an invisible realm that there's a Creator who made this world, and who is with me and for me, and even has a good purpose in the suffering."

Bobbitt also believes that faith helps you prioritize what's most important—character growth as a Christian to become like Jesus Christ and join Him in His sufferings. "Faith does so much for the future and for eternal hope," he said. "This isn't all there is. There's an entire eternity to be spent with God, enjoying Him in a world without pain and suffering. So it provides hope to draw you through the long time of suffering ahead."

But what exactly is faith? Hebrews 11:1 tells us that "faith is the assurance of things hoped for, the conviction of things not seen." Alan Wright said in his article "5 Lessons Cancer Patients Have Taught Me About Faith" that "hope and gratitude are the foundation of faith. Hope can stare down any diagnosis. Hope allows tears *and* laughter. Hope looks forward when all else tells us to give up. Optimism, on the other hand, is temporary, and is easily poked full of holes when life gets difficult. But faith, built on hope and gratitude, is enduring."[19]

Faith is also never stagnant. Faith changes. Faith is challenged, and it grows, particularly in the face of difficult times. Wright said, "A changing faith is a healthy faith."[20]

But a changing and a growing faith doesn't equal a life free from pain. In fact, Scripture tells us that we can be assured of times of trouble and pain. The Apostle James affirmed this truth when he said, "Count it all joy, my brothers, when you meet trials of various kinds, for you know that the testing of your faith produces steadfastness. And let steadfastness have its full effect, that you may be perfect and complete, lacking in nothing" (James 1:2-4). John 16:33 says, "I have said these things to you, that in me you may have peace. In the world you will have tribulation. But take heart; I have overcome the world."

Spiritual strength is critical in the fight against cancer. It can help you maintain a sense of hope and courage in the face of the disease. Melissa was diagnosed with squamous cell carcinoma, one of the most aggressive forms of head and neck cancer. Her diagnosis came in June 2020, and it took her on a spiritual journey she never expected. "I knew I was going to go through something really hard," she said. "But I also knew I would get through it. So I had that hope, but I had to keep fighting for that hope and really lean into the Lord and get to know the Holy Spirit in such an intimate and personal way. It sort of launched this gorgeous journey of discovering healing scriptures and walking through the life of Jesus and what He endured and all the pain He went through just to save my soul."

Melissa said she has no regrets. "It has just been really sweet," she said. "It probably sounds weird, but I would do it all again in a heartbeat just to know Jesus the way I know Him now. I would do it all again for that connection I have with Him."

Terry agrees. He was diagnosed with prostate cancer at the age of 80. Thankfully, it was confined to the prostate, but he underwent radiation treatment daily for eight weeks. The treatment affected him terribly. He began to wonder if dying was really all that bad. Radiation impacted his bladder, bowel, rectum, and stomach. While he is cancer-free today, he still lives with the ramifications of so much radiation. Despite all this, Terry said that getting cancer was one of the best things to happen to him.

"I thank the Lord for giving me cancer," he said. "I wouldn't have wanted to live without it. And people say, 'You're crazy,' but there's a reason it had such a purifying effect on me like nothing else ever has."

When going through cancer, you'll need your community of friends and family. But most importantly, you'll need the Lord. You cannot do this alone. When facing cancer, it's important to feed your faith, not your fears.

Perhaps it might be helpful to make peace—with yourself, with others, and with God. That's not meant to be morbid but rather to give you a place of serenity that passes all understanding.

As you make peace with yourself, remember that cancer is no respecter of persons. It doesn't care about your age, sex, faith, race, or anything else. It can happen to anyone, and it does.

Make peace with others. Forgive where necessary, and don't hold onto bitterness or wrath. That will allow you to carry fewer burdens into a very burdensome situation.

And make peace with God. This is not His punishment for you being a bad person. You may ask, "Why me, God?" And that's okay. Just don't allow yourself to get stuck in the question.

Perhaps ask God, "What can you teach me about You, me, or this situation that will allow me to grow?"

While your medical team is putting a care plan in place for your treatments, consider putting together your own spiritual care plan. I did this when I was first diagnosed. I determined that I would read from the Psalms while I was getting chemotherapy. I also wanted to take the time I had (many hours on end) during chemo to share Christ with other patients. I had a prayer journal, and a dear friend bought me a Bible Box that holds every card, gift, calendar and other memento that came along through the process. I was also certain that I'd spend hours in prayer.

If I'm honest, not much of that happened the way I had hoped. I did bring my Bible with me to the infusion room, but I was either too tired from the pre-meds to read for very long or I found myself people-watching instead of reading. I was fascinated by the sounds and the things the nurses were doing. I focused on them to pass the time. It seemed that every time I went to the infusion room ready to share Christ with someone, the people nearest me either were asleep during their infusions, had other guests with them, were engaged in conversation, or were wearing earbuds to block out the sounds or perhaps listen to music. I started a journal in my calendar, but that quickly faded as I got bored with it. I found it difficult to pray much at all during my cancer journey. Don't get me wrong, I did pray. But they were not the hours-long prayers of devotion I wanted for myself. Still, I felt close to the Lord, and my faith never wavered throughout that time. If anything, my faith grew by leaps and bounds.

For your own spiritual care plan, consider these things:

- *Pray.* It doesn't have to be long, intense prayers of worship, adoration, and supplication. I often asked God to heal me, and other times I was able to thank Him for the nursing and medical team He had put together on my behalf. And other times, I spent a few minutes praising Him for who He is.
- *Practice daily devotionals.* If you have the Bible app, there are tons of devotionals with various themes available, and it's free. Find a good book devotional that you can take with you to your treatments. If you have time and aren't too groggy, read one devotional per day.
- *Journal.* If you're like me and sometimes fall asleep when praying, write out your prayers. This is an excellent way to keep track of how God answers them. If you prefer, journal your thoughts. Writing your feelings down with pen and paper is very cathartic.
- *Read and meditate on Scripture.* You don't need to read an entire book of the Bible in a single sitting. Read a chapter or two. Read a verse or two if that's all you can handle. If you're new to the Bible, read one of the Gospels such as Mark or John. Find psalms that speak of God's healing power.
- *Find a safe space to talk, vent, and cry with others.* It's already been said but can't be said enough that you can't do this alone. Community and faith matter. Work on finding a community of believers who will provide you

a safe space to share from the heart. And allow others to pray for you. That, too, can be very healing.

- *Connect with activities.* Activities—exercise, music, spending time with friends or family—will lift your spirits. And be sure to laugh a lot!

- *Remember all the ways the Lord has been there for you.* Remember His faithfulness and His goodness. Remind yourself that He got you through tough times before, and He'll be faithful to do it again.

This was true of Hope. She was diagnosed with stage 0 breast cancer two weeks to the day after I received my diagnosis. We walked through this journey together, and I am so grateful for that time with her, although I hated what we were both going through. Hope had a lumpectomy and 20 rounds of radiation. She, too, is now cancer-free. As Hope and I reflected on our journey, she remembered that she is not in control of so many things but is thankful she knows the One who is. Hope shared this:

So all through my life there have been circumstances that I didn't have any control over. One was when my dad died when I was in college. I remembered that God got me through that. And then we were dealing with infertility and drugs and medicine and doctors. But God got us through that. God got us through the adoption process. It never dawned on me that He wouldn't get me through this. It was just a matter of like, "Okay, God. Here we go again." But I think because I saw how faithful He was in each prior big circumstance, I'm like, "Oh, He has me."

He did have Hope. And He has you too. And so do friends and family if you let them in. Remember, having a community and a strong faith in God will carry you through your darkest days.

Deeper Still ...

1. God made us for community. Having a community during the process of healing in your cancer journey is not only important but necessary. Have you found this to be true in your own experience? If so, explain what that looked like for you.

2. A community of people who are there for you can look different for everyone—a few trusted friends, a small group, a church family, or something else. What is the purpose of having a community? How did you find your community to be most helpful?

3. Feeling alone or isolated can be the worst part of the cancer journey. A listening ear, a physical touch, a caring heart, or simply the presence of another is vital. Knowing that someone is praying for you is the most encouraging. Have you had the privilege of coming alongside someone during their healing process? If so, describe what that was like for you.

4. How does God's Word define faith in Hebrews 11:1? What did you learn concerning faith and hope from the article by Alan Wright?

5. List the things to consider when putting together your own spiritual care plan. What would you find to be most beneficial?

6. From the several examples provided in this chapter of others who walked through their own cancer journey, note what they all had in common—their experience of drawing closer to Jesus and growing in their relationship with Him. Reflect on how He was there with you in your cancer journey or how you may have experienced His peace and presence. You might want to write out a prayer of thanksgiving.

Chapter 9

ONE MORE THING: THE GOOD NEWS

This book is intended to be a biblical guide to navigating life after cancer. Perhaps you've read it from cover to cover, including the Appendices in the back of the book. Maybe you've only hit one or two chapters that spoke to your current situation. Maybe you skipped Part I in order to get to the "good stuff" in Part II. However you've read it, I trust and pray that it's been a helpful guide and resource for your heart, mind, and soul. Wherever you are on your journey with cancer, I pray that this book has been an encouragement for you.

Perhaps you're reading this as a caregiver or a friend of someone who is going through cancer. I hope you, too, have been inspired and encouraged. Through all these things, it has been my greatest hope that everyone would see one theme running through this entire book—God is faithful.

Perhaps you know this faithful God. Maybe you've been walking with Him for years or maybe only for a short while. Wherever you are on your faith journey, I hope you have seen the goodness and faithfulness of God in your own life. And I pray that you see it in your cancer or after-cancer journey.

Perhaps you've never met the Jesus I speak of in this book. I'd like to take a moment to introduce Him to you. Since I've been sharing my cancer journey story, I'll continue with that theme. I'd like to tell you how I came to know the God who is merciful and full of love and tenderness, who held me in His arms when I needed Him most.

In my early 20s, I began dating a man who was a PK—a preacher's kid. He went to church every Sunday morning and Wednesday night without fail. Of course, I wanted to spend as much time with him as possible, so I started attending church with him. It was at this Southern Baptist church that I learned about the Jesus who died on the cross for me. I learned that Jesus paid the price for *my* sin on that cross so I could receive eternal life free from condemnation and judgment from God. As I learned more about this compassionate Jesus, I longed to know Him even more. One Sunday morning at the end of church, I went forward before the congregation and gave my life to Jesus Christ.

But in those moments, I am not entirely sure I was fully surrendered to Him. I still tried to do things my own way. I was stubborn at best and sinful at worst. I said and did all the things Christians are supposed to say and do, but I was incredibly selfish and, well, sinful. Not that I was trying to be perfect and sinless; I just wasn't living my life for Jesus. I was living it for myself, for my own gain and fortune. I went to church but fell into various temptations in my mid to late 20s. The consequences of my sins were the hardest to manage, but even then, I still didn't fully surrender to Jesus.

I walked the fence of being a Christian but not fully surrendering to His authority and His love for more than a decade. Working as a TV news journalist, I found myself across from the Pentagon in Washington, DC, on September 11, 2001, when our country was attacked. I heard the plane crash into the Pentagon, which caused me to freeze in fear. As a producer, I saw videos that most people have never seen—and I pray they never see—from raw footage taken that fateful day at Ground Zero. All that resulted in my continued state of paralyzing fear.

Ultimately, I left the Washington, DC, area to pursue a different form of journalism—print journalism—and relocated to Indianapolis, Indiana. I was as far from God at that point as I had ever been in my Christian walk. I was angry at what happened to our country, to New York, to the nearly 3,000 innocent people who died, and to me. Why did I have to go through what I went through? God couldn't—or wouldn't—answer the many questions I had. But God in His great mercy and love continued to pursue me.

I knew I needed to return to church and to the Lord. One Sunday I felt led by the Holy Spirit to visit a church not far from my home. It was in that Indianapolis church that I met my now husband, Kurt. Not long after we were married in 2004, I began down a path of extreme anger, depression, and anxiety. I was suicidal and made an attempt at my life about a year after our marriage. I was diagnosed with post-traumatic stress disorder from what I had experienced during and after 9/11. Glad to have a diagnosis, I began treatment for it and found myself healing in my mental well-being.

I was going to church again, but I found it difficult to connect with others because I felt that no one would understand what I had been through or my PTSD diagnosis. While I don't remember the exact year—it was 2014 or 2015—I fell into another deep depression. Despite being in a huge church, I continued to isolate myself, and being alone left me reeling. I made another attempt at suicide, and Kurt took me to the stress center at the hospital where I was ultimately admitted.

I was nearly strip-searched upon arrival to make sure I didn't have any weapons on me. I had to wear scrubs and hospital socks instead of my own clothes. I gave up my cell phone and had no other personal possessions with me except my toothbrush. I remember when the door slammed shut behind Kurt after we said our goodbyes that day. The sound reverberated through my brain as if I had just been locked in a prison cell. Perhaps it wasn't really that dramatic, but that's how I felt.

The gravity of the situation struck me, and I knew I needed to get right with myself and God. I needed to find healing because I knew suicide wasn't an option. The writer in me wanted to journal through this experience for posterity's sake and bring about healing, as writing had always done for me. However, the stress center didn't allow pens or pencils because you could use them to harm yourself or someone else. Instead, I was given a rubber pencil. I don't know if you've ever tried to write with a rubber pencil, but it's not as easy as it sounds.

I sat down at the table to write with my rubber pencil and realized I had nothing—no clothes, no shoes, no hairbrush, nothing from my home, nothing, not even a real pencil. As tears streamed down my cheeks, it suddenly dawned on me that what I did have was all that mattered. I had Jesus. I felt an overwhelming peace as I felt His presence descend on me in a way I had never experienced before. I felt love as I had never felt it. I saw the cross where He died for me, and I realized that this moment of being locked in a psychiatric hospital was one of the many reasons He had died for me. In that instant, I knew my life was forever changed, and I knew I would be okay. I had Jesus, and He was all I ever needed.

Once I was released, I promised myself that I would live for Jesus from that moment on. While I haven't done that perfectly, I have certainly given every part of myself to Him. I was invited by the wife of one of our church elders to do a book study. The years passed as she and I spent more and more time together. She taught me how to read and study the Bible. She taught me how to pray. She taught me how to surrender fully and what it means to fully surrender. I began to open my life to others and share my story. I began participating in our church's women's Bible study, and Kurt and I participated in a small group where we did life together while studying God's Word.

A few years after participating in our women's Bible study, I was asked to be a facilitator of that same study. I've been leading it for seven years now. Eventually, I was asked to lecture for our women's Bible study. I joined the Missions Team and used my writing gifts to create a monthly newsletter that goes out to our church body. I was asked to join the writing team, which includes women from our church who write our own curriculum for the women's Bible study. And Kurt and I now co-lead that small group we joined so many years ago. The Lord used what happened to me and turned it around for my good and for His glory. I'm still a sinner, but I'm learning and growing as a Christian, and I haven't "arrived" by any stretch of the imagination. I never will until He calls me to heaven. While the Lord has blessed me with much in so many different ways, Jesus is still all I need. And He's truly all I want. The rest is icing on the cake.

Every one of us is a sinner. The Bible says in Romans 3:23 that "all have sinned and fall short of the glory of God." We are all lost and in need of a Savior. And there is a Savior who loves you and wants to be in a relationship with you. John 3:16 tells us that "God so loved the world that He gave His only Son, that whoever believes in Him should not perish but have eternal life." That's how much Jesus loves you. Jesus died on the cross to pay the debt that we could never afford to pay ourselves. The Bible says in Romans 5:8, "But God shows his love for us in that while we were still sinners, Christ died for us." He willingly went to the cross to pay for the sins we have already committed and will still commit in the future.

One of the many beautiful parts of this is that when you commit your life to Jesus Christ, He welcomes you with open arms and remembers your sin no more. Psalm 103:11–12 promises, "For as high as the heavens are above the earth, so great is his steadfast love toward those who fear him; as far as the east is from the west, so far does he remove our transgressions from us." By surrendering to Jesus, you receive the free gift of eternal salvation that was paid through His death and resurrection. What that means is that when you die, you'll spend eternity in heaven with the God who created you, the God who loves you and chose you from before the foundation of the world.

So what do you have to do? Simply receive Jesus. You can't *do* anything to receive this free gift of salvation. You can't earn this salvation by being a good person. We are saved by faith through the grace of God alone. In other words, have faith in Jesus, confess that He is Lord, and then live your life accordingly and obediently. Romans 10:9 tells us that "if you confess with your mouth that Jesus is Lord and believe in your heart that God raised him from the dead, you will be saved."

Have you felt your heart stirring in affection toward Jesus as you've read this book? If so, I would like to encourage you to pray this prayer for yourself:

Dear God, I confess that I am a sinner in need of a Savior. I admit that I have made mistakes and have messed up terribly in the past. I confess that I am sinful at heart. Forgive me. Jesus, I ask you to come into my heart and cleanse me and make me clean by your blood. I need you and want to live my life for you. I surrender all to you right now. Fill me with your Holy Spirit so I can live for you. In Jesus's name. Amen.

If you just said that prayer, I want to say well done! Congratulations on accepting the invitation that Jesus extended to you. And welcome to the family of God! You are now the son or daughter of the King. Now I want you to tell someone about this monumental decision you've made. Share it with your spouse, your kids, your best friend. Find a Bible-believing church and tell them. Ask them to help guide you as you learn to walk by faith. Ask them to help you grow in your faith.

Once you've found a good, Bible-believing church, get a Bible (ask your pastor for a good translation). I encourage you to get a study Bible that will help answer a lot of questions as you read. If you're intimidated by reading the Bible, don't worry. You're not alone. I encourage you to start with one of the Gospels—Matthew, Mark, Luke, or John—found at the beginning of the New Testament. This will help you gain a foundational understanding of who Jesus is.

I also encourage you to be baptized. Baptism alone does not bring salvation, but it is a step of obedience on your spiritual journey. It is simply an outward expression of your faith and follows the example Jesus set for us when He was baptized.

Finally, cling to the Lord. If you're still in the middle of your cancer journey or struggling with the after-effects of that journey, ask God to meet you where you are. I promise you that He will.

Don't worry about doing everything perfectly. None of us are perfect as Christians. We still make mistakes, and we always will until Jesus comes back to make all things right. Being a Christian doesn't remove the fact that we are still sinners. We just know the One who washes away our sins.

Trust that the Lord loves you deeply. After all, He chose you. He has pursued you with an everlasting love. And He has a plan and a purpose for your life. Jeremiah 29:11 says, "For I know the plans I have for you, declares the Lord, plans for welfare and not for evil, to give you a future and a hope." Trust Him for the plans in your life, even the plans and purposes of your cancer journey.

If you have taken the step of trusting Jesus with your heart and your life, I would love to hear from you. I would love the opportunity to encourage you and pray that the Lord will bless you abundantly and provide healing for you or your friend or family member who is dealing with cancer.

And now I pray this prayer for you:

> *The LORD bless you and keep you; the LORD make his face to shine upon you and be gracious to you; the LORD lift up his countenance upon you and give you peace.*
>
> —Num. 6:24–26

Deeper Still …

1. How has this book been an encouragement to you?
2. Have you been motivated to share your own story of your cancer journey with others? If so, how will you implement that plan?
3. Learning of God's faithfulness in someone else's story should challenge us to look back at our own life. Record the ways you have seen God's faithfulness, and then praise Him with a heart of gratitude.

AN INTRODUCTION TO THE APPENDICES AND A STORY

Tana remembers exactly where she was when she received an urgent call from a doctor insisting that she take her daughter Haley to the children's hospital as soon as possible. While the word *leukemia* was mentioned, Tana didn't want to focus on that until she knew all the details. Haley, who was 12 at the time, was diagnosed with AML—acute myeloid leukemia. Once they received the diagnosis and were connected with the lead doctor, Tana remembers him saying, "I know that you all pray. We just need to pray for a miracle."

"We went from shock to sadness," Tana said. "Just a sadness that we've never known before. Life as we knew it had seemingly stopped."

Tana went into warrior mode to learn as much as she could about the disease that had the potential to take Haley's life. She wanted to make certain they were doing all they could to ensure Haley won the battle.

Haley was already wise beyond her years. She'd had some other medical challenges in her young life that required her to be stronger than a young girl should have to be. But she was full of life and joyful. She started experiencing some strange symptoms, including nausea, vomiting, passing out, and skin infections and blisters. They required doctors to take a closer look.

Upon receiving her diagnosis, she was admitted to the children's hospital immediately. She was told of the grueling and long battle she would face. To make matters worse, this was during the COVID-19 lockdowns. No one was allowed to visit her. Only one person, her mother, was allowed to be with her. Eventually, they allowed Tana and her middle daughter, Riley, to take turns staying with Haley in the hospital. That allowed both of them time to refresh, rest, and catch-up doing things around the house while ensuring that Haley was never alone during her cancer journey.

Haley stayed in the hospital for six months. Her chemotherapy treatments were both challenging and ghastly. She was told she had to have a stem cell transplant, and a donor was found outside the family. The family was so grateful for the soul who selflessly gave of himself to try to help a complete stranger. Haley's body had to be completely eradicated of the bad cells and be prepared for the new cells to come in and be effective and healthy. Haley was completely depleted. Her mother described her as near death, or flat.

Haley remembers being concerned about losing herself in the process. "When I first got the diagnosis, I was like, 'I'm never going to go back and be a normal teenager ever again. My skin is never going to be the same. My emotional cutoff is never going to be the same.' So it's like they're not kidding when you become a different person after something like this."

"That was the hardest part," Tana explained, "because you don't know if she's ever coming back."

Haley did come back. The transplant was a success, and although she continues to deal with graft versus host disease (GvHD), a systemic disorder that occurs when the graft's immune cells recognize the host as foreign and attack the recipient's body cells. Since the transplant, Haley's health has remained stable, and she has blossomed into a beautiful, joyful, mindful, caring teenager.

Because of GvHD, Haley is constantly being observed and requires a variety of labs and other tests to ensure that she remains healthy. While they work to maintain a healthy lifestyle and improvement of GvHD, there's never a guarantee, which can promote fear of recurrence.

"We might be back in the hospital next week," Tana said. "I don't know. That was a process of releasing that kind of, and I don't know if it was fear. I don't think it was fear, but it was more of a tentative response to normalcy because nothing is normal anymore. Yet the world still lives like normal. It moves on, and it wants you. It's beckoning you to reenter, but you can't because it's not the same for you."

So many of us as survivors expect to return to the way it used to be, but it will never be that way again. We are forever changed. That's not necessarily a bad thing. We have a new perspective on life and what's important to us. Bob Ash says that sitting with this new sense of normalcy is good for the soul. "I think sometimes we're in this notion that we should just get back to normal," he explained. "You don't even know what that is yet. So just when you talk about grief or anything else, we talk about any part of that survival process. Just don't be in a hurry because you need to take time to figure out what this new normal is. And it's not going to be a quick thing."

Eric Bobbitt reminds us that cancer teaches us that a lot doesn't matter; only a few things matter. "You have to rebuild your life on things that actually matter," he explained. He encourages cancer survivors to take the time to ponder what matters and how to rebuild their life around those things.

You can find new life and meaning after your own cancer journey. Some people say that cancer was a wake-up call and allowed them to reassess their own lives. Perhaps you could do the same. Seek spiritual and emotional support in your after-cancer care. Keep a journal and write down what is giving you meaning in your life after cancer. Some people help themselves heal by helping others heal. Give your life new meaning by helping others overcome in their cancer journey.

Perhaps your greatest battle in navigating life after cancer is the fear of recurrence. This is common among nearly every cancer survivor, regardless of the type or severity of that cancer.

There is always the unknown, but Tana says there is a way to combat the fear of recurrence.

> Lean into God's face. Fill the reservoir of your soul, your mind with truth, and pray that He would give you an eternal perspective because nothing is promised beyond this moment that we're living. And there could be a life-altering event that happens to

any one of us 10 minutes from now. So you have to have an eternal perspective of the hope that we are sure of. Life is but a vapor, as Scripture tells us. And so to cling to the promises of truth, of hope, and of eternity, that's the only way you can navigate life after cancer. Otherwise, there would be the temptation to either live in fear, worry, or self-pity, none of which the Lord wants for us.

In the pages that follow are several resources for you and your loved ones. Discover the character of God by learning of His attributes and who He is. Find out some of the many promises of God for you, His beloved. Explore who you are in Christ and then read various scriptures on the topics of grief and fear. I pray that these are helpful to you.

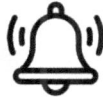

ACKNOWLEDGMENTS

A very special thanks to my Lord and Savior Jesus Christ without whom none of this would be possible. Thank you for saving me, and thank you for healing me.

A very special thanks to my prayer team who has been on this journey with me from the very beginning and have faithfully prayed over every aspect of this book project. Thanks to Becky, Patty, Diane, Tana, Deb, Traci, Arlene, Diana, Kristina, Monique, Lori, and Kate.

A very special thanks to my mother, Margarete, who supported me through this project and cared for me so well during my cancer journey.

Special thanks to Patty and Lori without whom this book wouldn't be what it is. Thank you for your giftedness and wisdom in the scriptures and for helping others to go deeper still.

Appendix A
THE CHARACTER OF GOD

INCOMMUNICABLE	COMMUNICABLE
These attributes reside in God alone and cannot be passed on to us.	*These attributes find their complete expression in God, while humans can experience them in limited form.*

SELF-EXISTENT: God was not made. He has no origin. There is nothing upon which God depends for His existence.

SELF-SUFFICIENT: Within Himself, God is able to act. He has a voluntary relationship to everything He has made. He may choose to use us but doesn't need us to accomplish His will.

HOLY: God is totally separated from evil, completely pure, morally excellent. He cannot be otherwise.

ALL-WISE: God cannot make a mistake. He has an unlimited ability to correctly apply his all-encompassing knowledge. He achieves perfect ends by perfect means.

IMMUTABLE: God is limitless, boundless, and measureless.

INFINITE: God is limitless, boundless, and measureless.

ETERNAL: God has no beginning or end. He is everlasting, timeless.

TRANSCENDENT: God's existence is totally apart from His creatures or creation. He is far above the created universe.

INCOMPREHENSIBLE: God is beyond our understanding, unsearchable. It is only by self-disclosure that we can understand or know anything about Him.

LOVE: By His very essence, His very nature, God is love. It is an active, unconditional, demonstrative love.

JUST: God is completely fair in all His actions. There is no injustice with God.

GOOD: God is benevolent and kind. He is the source of all good.

WRATHFUL: Because He is pure and completely separated from evil, God hates unrighteousness. He is always angry with sin.

MERCIFUL: God is actively compassionate in confronting human misery and guilt. It is an expression of His goodness.

SOVEREIGN: God reigns supremely and is in control of all things.

OMNIPOTENT: God is all-powerful. By choice, He is able to bring about anything. He has unlimited power, force, and authority.

OMNISCIENT: God is all-knowing. He knows all the past, the present, the future, and all possibilities.

OMNIPRESENT: God is everywhere present in all the universe at all times.

LONG-SUFFERING: God chooses to put up with humankind. His just anger is slow to be kindled against those who fail to listen to His warnings or obey His instructions.

FAITHFUL: God is totally steadfast to what He has spoken. He is always true to His promises because He does not change and cannot lie.

TRUTHFUL: Integrity is inherent in God's nature. He is always accurate, genuine, exact, and precise.

Appendix B

THE PROMISES OF GOD

These are just a few of the thousands of promises of God to you in His written Word. Trust in the promises of God as you navigate life during or after cancer. He is faithful; surely, He will do it.

1. **God promises to strengthen you.**

   For this reason *I bow my knees before the Father, from whom every family in heaven and on earth is named, that according to the riches of his glory he may grant you to be strengthened with power through his Spirit in your inner being.*

   —Eph. 3:14–16

2. **God promises to give you rest.**

   Then Jesus said, "Come to me, all of you who are weary and carry heavy burdens, and I will give you rest. Take my yoke upon you. Let me teach you, *because I am humble and gentle at heart, and you will find rest for your souls. For my yoke is easy to bear, and the burden I give you is light."*

   —Matt. 11:28–30 (NLT)

3. **God promises to take care of all your needs.**

And this same God who takes care of me will supply all your needs from his glorious riches, which have been given to us in Christ Jesus.

—Phil. 4:19 (NLT)

4. **God promises to answer your prayers.**

Ask, and it will be given to you; seek, and you will find; knock, and it will be opened to you.

—Matt. 7:7

5. **God promises to work everything out for your good.**

And we know that God causes everything to work together for the good of those who love God and are called according to his purpose for them.

—Rom. 8:28 (NLT)

6. **God promises to be with you.**

I will not fail you or abandon you. This is my command—be strong and courageous! Do not be afraid or discouraged. For the LORD your God is with you wherever you go.

—Josh. 1:5, 9 (NLT)

7. **God promises to protect you.**

This I declare about the LORD: He alone is my refuge, my place of safety; he is my God, and I trust him.
—Ps. 91:2 (NLT)

8. **God promises freedom from sin.**

But if we confess our sins to him, he is faithful and just to forgive us our sins and to cleanse us from all wickedness.
—1 John 1:9 (NLT)

So if the Son sets you free, you will be free indeed.
—John 8:36

9. **God promises that nothing can separate you from Him.**

For I am sure that neither death nor life, nor angels nor rulers, nor things present nor things to come, nor powers, nor height nor depth, nor anything else in all creation, will be able to separate us from the love of God in Christ Jesus our Lord.
—Rom. 8:38–39

10. **God promises you everlasting life.**

For God so loved the world, that he gave his only Son, that whoever believes in him should not perish but have eternal life.
—John 3:16

Appendix C

SCRIPTURES FOR DEALING WITH GRIEF

salm 55:16–17: *But I call to God, and the L*ORD *will save me. Evening and morning and at noon I utter my complaint and moan, and He hears my voice.*

Matthew 11:28–30: *Come to me, all who labor and are heavy laden, and I will give you rest. Take my yoke upon you, and learn from me, for I am gentle and lowly in heart, and you will find rest for your souls. For my yoke is easy, and my burden is light.*

Isaiah 66:13: *As one whom his mother comforts, so I will comfort you; you shall be comforted in Jerusalem.*

Psalm 23:1–4: *The L*ORD *is my shepherd; I shall not want. He makes me lie down in green pastures. He leads me beside still waters. He restores my soul. He leads me in paths of righteousness for His name's sake. Even though I walk through the valley of the shadow of death, I will fear no evil, for you are with me; your rod and your staff, they comfort me.*

Isaiah 41:9–10: *You whom I took from the ends of the earth, and called from its farthest corners, saying to you, "You are my servant, I have chosen you and not cast you off"; fear not, for I am with you; be not dismayed, for I am your God; I will strengthen you, I will help you, I will uphold you with my righteous right hand.*

Lamentations 3:21–23: *But this I call to mind, and therefore I have hope. The steadfast love of the LORD never ceases; His mercies never come to an end; they are new every morning; great is your faithfulness.*

Psalm 143:8: *Let me hear in the morning of your steadfast love, for in you I trust. Make me know the way I should go, for to you I lift up my soul.*

2 Corinthians 1:3–4: *Blessed be the God and Father of our Lord Jesus Christ, the Father of mercies and God of all comfort, who comforts us in all our affliction, so that we may be able to comfort those who are in any affliction, with the comfort with which we ourselves are comforted by God.*

Revelation 21:4–5: *He will wipe away every tear from their eyes, and death shall be no more, neither shall there be mourning, nor crying, nor pain anymore, for the former things have passed away. And he who was seated on the throne said, "Behold I am making all things new." Also he said, "Write this down, for these words are trustworthy and true."*

1 Peter 1:3–4: *Blessed be the God and Father of our Lord Jesus Christ! According to his great mercy, he has caused us to be born again to a living hope through the resurrection of Jesus Christ from the dead, to an inheritance that is imperishable, undefiled, and unfading, kept in heaven for you.*

Appendix D

SCRIPTURES ON FEAR

Psalm 46:1–3: *God is our refuge and strength, a very present help in trouble. Therefore, we will not fear though the earth gives way, though the mountains be moved into the heart of the seas, though its waters roar and foam, though the mountains tremble at its swelling.*

Psalm 56:3–4: *When I am afraid, I put my trust in you. In God, whose word I praise, in God I trust; I shall not be afraid. What can flesh do to me?*

Mark 9:24: *Immediately the father of the child cried out and said, "I believe; help my unbelief!"*

1 Peter 5:6–7: *Humble yourselves, therefore, under the mighty hand of God so that at the proper time he may exalt you, casting all your anxieties on him, because he cares for you.*

Romans 8:31: *If God is for us, who can be against us?*

Joshua 1:9: *Have I not commanded you? Be strong and courageous. Do not be frightened, and do not be dismayed, for the* LORD *your God is with you wherever you go.*

Romans 8:38–39: *For I am sure that neither death nor life, nor angels nor rulers, nor things present nor things to come, nor powers, nor height nor depth, nor anything else in all creation, will be able to separate us from the love of God in Christ Jesus our Lord.*

Proverbs 3:5–6: *Trust in the* LORD *with all your heart, and do not lean on your own understanding. In all your ways acknowledge him, and he will make straight your paths.*

Philippians 4:6: *Do not be anxious about anything, but in everything by prayer and supplication with thanksgiving let your requests be made known to God.*

John 14:27: *Peace I leave with you; my peace I give to you. Not as the world gives do I give to you. Let not your hearts be troubled, neither let them be afraid.*

Isaiah 26:3–4: *You keep him in perfect peace whose mind is stayed on you, because he trusts in you. Trust in the* LORD *forever, for the* LORD GOD *is an everlasting rock.*

ENDNOTES

1. Heather L. Van Epps, "Seeing Red: Coping with Anger During Cancer," Cure 11, no. 2 (2012), https://www.curetoday.com/view/seeing-red-coping-with-anger-during-cancer.

2. Van Epps.

3. Tim Challies, *Seasons of Sorrow* (Zondervan, 2022), 59.

4. Ray Stedman, *Ray Stedman Ministries*, 2023, www.raystedman.org.

5. Alan D. Wolfelt, PhD, "Coping with Cancer," *Coping with Cancer*, March/April 2019, https://copingmag.com/the-grief-and-mourning-of-cancer/.

6. "Seeking Help and Support for Grief and Loss," *American Cancer Society*, https://www.cancer.org/cancer/end-of-life-care/grief-and-loss/depression-and-complicated-grief.html.

7. Natasha Carlson, "Cancer Ghosting Is an Unfortunate Reality," *Cure*, January 26, 2023, https://www.curetoday.com/view/-cancer-ghosting-is-an-unfortunate-reality.

8. Kerry McAvoy, "Accept People Will Come and Go," *Kerry McAvoy PhD,* n.d., https://kerrymcavoyphd.com/how-being-ghosted-improved-my-life/.

9. Lysa TerKeurst, *Good Boudaries and Goodbyes* (Nelson Books, 2022), XVI.

10. TerKeurst, XVI.

11. TerKeurst, 17.

12. Josh Squires, "Marital Intimacy Is More Than Sex," *Desiring God*, March 2, 2016. https://www.desiringgod.org/articles/ marital-intimacy-is-more-than-sex.

13. Squires.

14. Squires.

15. Squires.

16. Squires.

17. Timothy Keller, *Walking with God Through Pain and Suffering* (Riverhead Books, 2013), 120.

18. Keller, 190–192.

19. Alan Wright, "5 Lessons Cancer Patients Have Taught Me About Faith," *Baylor Scott & White Health*, May 14, 2019, https://www.bswhealth.com/blog/5-lessons-cancer-patients-have-taught-me-about-faith.

20. Wright.